Sustainable Development Goals Series

The **Sustainable Development Goals Series** is Springer Nature's inaugural cross-imprint book series that addresses and supports the United Nations' seventeen Sustainable Development Goals. The series fosters comprehensive research focused on these global targets and endeavours to address some of society's greatest grand challenges. The SDGs are inherently multidisciplinary, and they bring people working across different fields together and working towards a common goal. In this spirit, the Sustainable Development Goals series is the first at Springer Nature to publish books under both the Springer and Palgrave Macmillan imprints, bringing the strengths of our imprints together.

The Sustainable Development Goals Series is organized into eighteen subseries: one subseries based around each of the seventeen respective Sustainable Development Goals, and an eighteenth subseries, "Connecting the Goals", which serves as a home for volumes addressing multiple goals or studying the SDGs as a whole. Each subseries is guided by an expert Subseries Advisor with years or decades of experience studying and addressing core components of their respective Goal.

The SDG Series has a remit as broad as the SDGs themselves, and contributions are welcome from scientists, academics, policymakers, and researchers working in fields related to any of the seventeen goals. If you are interested in contributing a monograph or curated volume to the series, please contact the Publishers: Zachary Romano [Springer; zachary.romano@springer.com] and Rachael Ballard [Palgrave Macmillan; rachael.ballard@palgrave.com].

Pranitha Maharaj
Editor

Navigating Ageing in South Africa

Interdisciplinary Perspectives

palgrave
macmillan

Editor
Pranitha Maharaj
School of Built Environment and Development Studies
University of KwaZulu-Natal
Durban, South Africa

ISSN 2523-3084 ISSN 2523-3092 (electronic)
Sustainable Development Goals Series
ISBN 978-981-97-9087-6 ISBN 978-981-97-9088-3 (eBook)
https://doi.org/10.1007/978-981-97-9088-3

This Palgrave Macmillan imprint is published by the registered company Springer Nature Singapore Pte Ltd.
The registered company address is: 152 Beach Road, #21-01/04 Gateway East, Singapore 189721, Singapore

Contents

Notes on Contributors

Shanaaz Dunn is the data manager in the Developmental, Capable and Ethical State (DCES) division at the Human Sciences Research Council (HSRC). She holds a PhD in Population Studies from the University of KwaZulu-Natal (UKZN). Before joining the HSRC, Shanaaz worked as the Research Manager for the DSI/NRF South African Research Chair Initiative (SARChI) in Economic Development at UKZN. Her research interests are broadly in the field of demography and population studies.

Nicolas Farina is an experienced dementia researcher and co-investigator on the STRiDE project. His work focuses on improving outcomes in people living with dementia and their carers and includes understanding factors associated with quality of life in people with dementia and addressing dementia-related stigma in the community.

Viloshin Govender is a senior lecturer at the School of Built Environment and Development Studies, University of KwaZulu-Natal, Durban. He holds a PhD in Architecture. His research involves working with marginalized communities, especially those in informal settlements, using drone technologies and community collaboration to create solutions that form a bottom-up approach. He is also a practising architect with research interests that include resilient cities, building adaptability, and how insurgency affects city planning.

Roxanne Jacobs is a researcher at the Alan J. Flisher Centre for Public Mental Health at the University of Cape Town, South Africa. She joined the STRiDE network as an early career researcher for the South African component. Her work includes research on stigma and dementia, ageing, and elder abuse.

Siyamthanda Jordaan is a researcher at the School of Built Environment and Development Studies. He holds an Honours degree in Population Studies from the University of KwaZulu-Natal and is currently pursuing his Master's degree which focuses on ageing. His research interests include ageing, sexual and reproductive health, development, and social policy.

Pranitha Maharaj is a professor at the School of Built Environment and Development Studies, University of KwaZulu-Natal, Durban, South Africa. She holds a PhD from the London School of Hygiene and Tropical Medicine in the United Kingdom. She has worked extensively in the field of demography and has published a number of articles on ageing in Africa.

Themba Mgwaba is senior lecturer in Population Studies at the School of Built Environment and Development Studies, University of KwaZulu-Natal, Durban. His teaching and research areas include ageing, HIV and AIDS, food security, migration, and urbanization. He has a special interest in HIV prevention and treatment amongst young people and students.

Sunday Israel Oyebamiji is a researcher and lecturer at the University of KwaZulu-Natal, South Africa. He holds a PhD in International Relations from the University of KwaZulu-Natal. He has an educational background in strategic studies and international relations and is committed to interdisciplinary research and teaching. His teaching and research interests include economic history and development studies, political science, and international relations.

Benjamin Roberts is a research director in the Developmental, Capable and Ethical State (DCES) programme at the Human Sciences Research Council (HSRC) and a visiting fellow at the Institute of Social and Economic Research (ISER) at Rhodes University. He holds a PhD in Social Policy and Labour Studies from Rhodes University. He has coordinated the South African Social Attitudes Survey (SASAS) series since its inception in 2003, with the 20th annual round of surveying completed in late 2023. His areas of expertise include attitudinal measurement and social change, poverty and inequality, subjective well-being, and quality of life.

Marguerite Schneider is an emeritus associate professor from the University of Cape Town and led the STRiDE project component in South Africa. She has extensive experience in applied disability studies and public mental health research. She has published on disability measurement, the intersection of disability, poverty and social protection, and public mental health.

Sachin Sewpersad is a researcher at the School of Built Environment and Development Studies, University of KwaZulu-Natal, Durban, South Africa. He has a Master's degree in Population Studies from the University of KwaZulu-Natal. His research and academic interests include ageing populations, migration, human environments, and other environmental processes.

List of Figures

List of Tables

1

Understanding Ageing in South Africa

Pranitha Maharaj

Abstract South Africa has one of the most rapidly growing ageing populations in Africa. While the population of South Africa is youthful, people aged 60 years and over increasingly constitute a proportionally larger share of the total population. The ageing of the population in South Africa is occurring in the context of widespread poverty and a host of other problems. As people grow older, they are more likely to experience physical decline and a range of health ailments, which is likely to increase demands on health systems. An ageing population is likely to have far-reaching implications for the country, not least as a major driver of population growth but also placing demands on resources and services. This chapter profiles the situation of older people in South Africa. Older people face a number of challenges, but they make a valuable contribution to the country.

P. Maharaj (✉)
School of Built Environment and Development Studies, University of KwaZulu-Natal, Durban, South Africa
e-mail: maharajp7@ukzn.ac.za

P. Maharaj (ed.), *Navigating Ageing in South Africa*, Sustainable Development Goals Series, https://doi.org/10.1007/978-981-97-9088-3_1

Keywords Ageing • Overview • Definition • Challenges • South Africa

Introduction

This book explores the situation of older people in South Africa. South Africa is an important case study for a number of reasons. It has one of the most rapidly ageing populations in the continent. While half of the population of South Africa is younger than 35, more people than ever before are living longer, and as of late more people are living into their seventies and beyond. It is important to note that projections suggest that the population is becoming increasingly older, and in the future, the current large number of young people will eventually progress to an older population. Over the past few decades, life expectancy has made significant gains as a result of range of interventions, both public as well as medical, and is an indication of economic progress. However, life expectancy took a slight knock as a result of the global COVID-19 pandemic with the estimated total life expectancy at birth dropping from 64.7 years in 2019 to 61.7 years in 2021, followed by a slight increase to 62.8 years in 2022 (Statistics South Africa, 2022). From a demographic and public health perspective, the massive increase in the number of people reaching older age is viewed as a success story, indicating medical, social, and economic advancement, but it also presents tremendous challenges for the country.

The population is likely to remain youthful but projections suggest that the number of older people is likely to increase significantly in the next few decades. The current demographic situation provides a unique window of opportunity to create and improve systems and institutions to respond to the maturing population in the longer term (Aboderin & Gelfand, 2019). In addition, all individuals deserve attention from governments and societies to promote their well-being and participation. Protection of the rights of older people is enshrined in the Constitution of the Republic of South Africa, 1996. There is a recognition of the vital role that is played by older people in the country and the Older Persons Act of 2006 protects them in law. However, ageing of the population is occurring in the context of widespread poverty, high levels of crime, changing household structures, a heavy disease burden, as well as infrastructural and service delivery challenges. Some strides have been made to respond effectively to the challenge of population ageing, but it will require a more detailed understanding of the situation of the older population in South Africa. This book attempts to fill the gaps that exist by exploring the social realities of navigating ageing in South Africa.

Overview of Ageing

Like most of Africa, South Africa has a relatively youthful country but is currently experiencing a growth in the number and proportion of older people in the population. Resultantly, older people constitute a large proportion of the population. Recent estimates suggest that the country has a population of approximately 62 million people and has one of the fastest growing ageing populations in Africa, with more than one in eight persons aged 60. The absolute number of persons aged 60 years and over has increased steadily from 4.1 million in 2011 to 5.6 million in 2022 and some projections suggest that the older population will continue to grow steadily over the next few decades (Statistics South Africa, 2023). In 2022, older persons aged 60 years and over constituted nearly 9.2% of the population and this is projected to grow to over 15% of the population in 2050 (Statistics South Africa, 2023). The population aged 60 years and older rose from 1.1% for the period 2002–2003 to 3% for the period 2019–2020 (Statistics South Africa, 2019). As fertility levels steadily decline and longevity continues to increase, the older population is expected to grow substantially over the next few decades. Projections show that the older population will continue to increase and by 2030 there will be approximately 7 million elderly persons in South Africa (Statistics South Africa, 2011). This suggests that the population is increasingly becoming older, indicating that in the future older people are likely to occupy a larger share of the population. It is also worth noting that at present the oldest old (those age 80 and over) constitute a small segment of the older population but this is also likely to change in the future.

Old age is widely acknowledged as inevitable and the last developmental stage in the lifecycle, characterised by physical, psychological, and, also, social changes. Until relatively recently, the older population has not received much attention in South Africa but this is slowly changing. There is no single, universally accepted definition of old age. Often the measures used to determine who is, or is not old, vary considerably, sometimes from region to region. In developed countries, chronological age is given far greater importance than in developing countries. The age of retirement, usually 60 or 65 years, is regarded as the onset of old age. In Africa, the use of chronological age—which is sometimes not even known—is problematic especially given that a large share of older people live in rural areas and may not even know their exact date of birth. In addition, a large number of older people are neither in formal employment nor entitled to formal retirement or its benefits. Other social constructions are therefore assigned greater prominence in trying to understand the process of ageing in Africa including physical appearances. For some, physical characteristics like wrinkles and grey hair are viewed as defining characteristics of older people. For others, the commencement of old age is seen to begin at that point in life when people, because of physical decline, are no longer able to independently perform their work and family roles. In this case, functional rather than chronological age is viewed as a more robust indicator of ageing. According to the functional definition, *the aged* refers to those who are unable to fully support or take care of themselves, and who also display the characteristics of being old (Roebuck, 1979). However, functional age does not always correspond to chronological age. For example, it has been pointed out that two persons may share the same chronological age of 60 years but they may differ immensely in their functional capabilities. Thus, people younger than 60 years may be widely regarded as old because they share the same physical and health conditions as people 60 years and older. In addition, some 60-year-olds may share the same physical and mental abilities as 30-year-olds. It also happens that people who are older than this chronological age do not want to be identified as 'old'. There has been widespread criticism of the 'one size fits all' approach that sets old age at a fixed chronological age, arguing it is not realistic. It has become increasing evident that there is substantial heterogeneity in the older cohort. In addition to having widely varying abilities, there is also likely to be considerable diversity by gender, class, ethnicity, and nationality. In South Africa, an older person is used to refer to someone aged 60 years and over. However, the Older Persons Act, No. 13 of 2006 initially defined an older person as someone who, in the case of a male, is 65 years of age or older and, in the case of a female, 60 years of age or older. It was only after 2008 that there was a harmonisation of age for men and women and it is now 60 years for both men and women.

The rapid ageing of the population is also occurring in the context of high levels of poverty and inequality. South Africa is classified as an upper-middle income country, with a ranking on the human development index of 109, with a score of 0.71 (United Nations, 2022). Absolute poverty is widespread, with almost 18.2 million people living in extreme poverty (those living under $1.90 per day) and there are significant levels of inequality with a Gini coefficient of 63 (Ngubane et al., 2023), making South Africa the most unequal country in the world, a legacy of apartheid's racially biased policies, which classified the population into four race groups: white, Indian (or Asian), coloured (of mixed heritage), and black (or African). This classification was meant to separate the various groups in every aspect of daily life. These discriminatory policies have left behind a legacy of huge inequalities, with the impact being felt most severely by Africans, including the oldest in the population. Africans constitute the majority of the population and even today the legacy of apartheid continues to be felt most severely by older African people. Education among older Africans remains very low, with almost 58% having less than primary school education (Statistics South Africa, 2023). In addition, while there have been significant improvements in access to basic services like housing, water, and sanitation, older Africans still lag behind the other groups. In 2021, almost 66% of older Africans had access to piped water compared to over 90% for other groups. Similarly, in 2021, 81% of older Africans had access to improved sanitation compared to nearly universal access of the other older groups (Statistics South Africa, 2023).

Older people are widely recognised as one of the most affected by poverty. In South Africa, more than 40% of older people live in the poorest conditions (Solanki et al., 2019). Poverty is more prominent in rural areas which are more likely to experience economic deprivation and resource scarcity. A key feature of ageing in South Africa is the disproportionate number of the older population living in rural areas. Rural areas are inhabited mainly by older people as a result of increasing migration and urbanisation. In South Africa there are distinct differences by geographical region. Often urban areas are characterised by much better resources and services than rural areas. At older ages, women constitute a much greater proportion than men, suggesting a feminisation of the older population. The higher proportion of women at the older ages is related to their longer life expectancy. Women tend to live much longer than men but they face their own unique set of challenges.

AIDS has also had a devastating effect on the country. The levels of HIV prevalence among all groups remains stubbornly high and older people are not unaffected. With more than 8 million people living with the virus, South Africa has one of the highest rates in the world. In South Africa, AIDS disproportionately impacted adults in the prime working age groups, altering the usual patterns of mortality and morbidity. The increasing availability of anti-retroviral drugs means that much more people with HIV are now living to later ages, which has major implications in terms of their health needs, particularly as the risk of chronic diseases of lifestyle increases as they get older. As a result of HIV and AIDS, older people and particularly women also have had to take on additional responsibilities that they had not planned on. They find themselves saddled with the duty of providing care and support for family members residing in their households (Baloyi, 2015).

South Africa is still recovering from the aftereffects of the emergence and rapid spread of the severe acute respiratory syndrome (SARS) coronavirus since the first case was discovered in March 2020. While the entire population is at risk of becoming infected, early evidence showed that older persons had a heightened risk of severe illness when infected (NICD, 2020). The risk of severe illness and mortality increased significantly with age due to reduced immunity as well as the presence of one or more pre-existing chronic conditions (NICD, 2020). As the number of infections spread quickly in the country, the government implemented strict national lockdown measures including stay-at-home orders, the closure of non-essential businesses, and limitations on travel and movement. Although the intention of these stringent early measures was to preserve life, they had a profound effect on mental health and emotional well-being which is likely to have long-term consequences.

Challenges of Ageing

Even though people in South Africa are living longer than they did in the past, this does not translate into better health for all. As people grow older they are more likely to face a range of health challenges that are associated with the ageing process. They are at great risk of non-communicable diseases such as cardiovascular diseases, diabetes, cancer, and chronic respiratory diseases. The three most frequent health conditions among older people are hypertension, diabetes, and asthma (Statistics South Africa, 2023). Older people are more likely to develop chronic conditions than younger people because their immune systems weaken significantly with age. As people age, they are at increased risk of not only experiencing chronic conditions but also co-morbidities (more than one chronic condition), which can complicate treatment and consequently the management of their health. As a result, some older adults are prescribed multiple medications that may interact with each other. In their study, Solanki et al. (2019) found that adults aged 60 years and over are much more likely than under-60s to develop chronic conditions.

As people age, they are less likely to engage in physical activities. Physical inactivity increases the risk of developing conditions such as coronary heart disease, diabetes, stroke, hypertension, and depression. A study done in low and middle-income countries including South Africa found that older working adults were clearly more active than those who were not working or were retired/too old to work (Gaskin & Orellana, 2018). This study suggests that physical work-related activity (e.g., use of transport to and from work, and employment-related physical activity) is not replaced with any other activity (e.g., leisure time activities) for older adults who are otherwise not working. As people age, they are more likely to experience physical decline resulting in frailty which can lead to heightened risks of falls, disability, and hospitalisation.

Disability increases in frequency with age; with 53.2% of elderly people aged 85 years and older reported to having disability in South Africa (Statistics South Africa, 2022). Older people are more likely to experience disabilities, affecting their functionality, and as a result, compromising their ability to perform basic daily activities independently, like cooking, bathing, and walking. The ability to carry out fundamental tasks that are necessary for daily living is frequently hampered by functional decline and physical reliance that come with ageing. A national population-based survey of 50 years and over found that physical inactivity and lower quality of life were associated with functional disability with women having a higher disability prevalence (Phaswana-Mafuya et al., 2013). Difficulties in performing basic daily activities of living are more common among older adults, negatively impacting their health and quality of life, and consequently increasing their reliance on care. People living with disabilities have a heightened risk of malnutrition, depression, loneliness, as well as frequent hospitalisation (Yaya et al., 2020).

Cognitive conditions like depression, anxiety, and dementia are also fairly common among older people. A nationally representative household survey conducted in South Africa reported the lifetime prevalence rate of major depression to be 9.7% with a significant association for women (Tomlinson et al., 2009). However, the 2008 SAGE study, a national population-based cross-sectional study of older South Africans, reported a 4% 12-month prevalence of symptom-based depression (Peltzer & Phaswana-Mafuya, 2013). Depression is not uncommon among older people with higher levels reported in rural than urban areas. One study found that the prevalence of major depression is 27% in rural settings and 25.2% in urban settings (Padayachey et al., 2017). The risk of dementia also increases with age. Dementia is a broad term used to describe a progressive or chronic neurodegenerative condition, largely impacting cognitive areas such as memory, language, orientation, and executive functioning (WHO, 2019). A study conducted in rural KwaZulu-Natal suggests that the prevalence of dementia may be as high as 13% for older adults. In this study, ageing was the primary risk factor for dementia, with the risk of dementia in those aged < 80 years almost double compared to those aged 60–69 years (Mfene & Pillay, 2023).

Unlike many infectious illnesses that are curable, the management of dementia is costly and requires long-term care and support.

As more people transition to old age, they are more likely to experience sensory impairments, such as hearing and vision loss. Some may experience dental issues, including tooth loss, gum disease, and oral infections. Their dental problems may also put them at risk of malnutrition. Older people may also be at risk of malnutrition due to factors such as reduced appetite, difficulty in preparing meals, and inadequate access to nutritious food. In some parts of South Africa, food insecurity remains a major challenge. Malnutrition can exacerbate other health conditions and lead to weight loss, muscle wasting, and impaired immune function. Many older people in South Africa find themselves living in poverty, which can affect their access to healthy food, adequate housing, and healthcare services. Social inequality can also contribute to disparities in health outcomes among different population groups of older people.

Older people are also likely to experience isolation either because they are living alone or due to a lack of social ties. Older adults who are in poor health are also less likely to participate in community activities. In the Western Cape, a study of the elderly at a community centre in a township found high levels of loneliness as well as social and emotional isolation among the elderly (Chigali et al., 2002). Loneliness refers to a subjective negative feeling characterised by both emotional and social isolation (Ntozini & Abdullahi, 2021). Social isolation is a consequence of a feeling of detachment from a social network or community, whereas emotional isolation stems from the death or absence of an attachment figure like a spouse (Chigali et al., 2002). The inability to participate in normal relationships and activities results in increasing separation from mainstream society and eventually social exclusion (Walsh et al., 2017). In general, studies suggest that individuals who have more frequent social interactions tend to experience a higher sense of well-being. Older people tend to feel much happier if they are around other people, they participate in social activities and have greater opportunities for social interaction (Ntozini & Abdullahi, 2021). However, this is likely to become less frequent as a result of their deteriorating health, and mobility. Their health condition may also be exacerbated by social isolation, limited mobility accompanied by loss of independence, and the grief associated with the loss of social interactions.

Thus, the longer people live, the greater the demand on health services. Access to healthcare services is often a major challenge for older people, especially for those in remote or rural areas as well as those with mobility issues. The majority of older people live in rural areas and struggle to get to healthcare facilities due to a lack of affordable and accessible transport. Most of the population in South Africa rely on the public sector which is state funded. However, they still have to cover out-of-pocket expenses for their medication which may be a significant barrier for the older people who are dependent on social grants. Geographical location may also influence access to health care. Older people living in rural or remote areas often experience difficulties in accessing health services due to long distances and lack of transportation. A number of studies reported that the location of health facilities is not convenient for older patients (Mussie et al., 2022; Schatz et al., 2018). Since health services are usually located some distance from their place of residences, older adults with mobility issues do not receive appropriate support and care. In order not to face the long distances to health facilities, older persons sometimes postpone their visit until they experience more severe health conditions or symptoms, which warrant them spending the money to get private transportation to the health centre (Schatz et al., 2018).

Public healthcare facilities are often overcrowded, leading to long waiting times for services. Older people with health complications may struggle to wait for extended periods, especially as they have to arrive early at the health facilities in order to ensure that they are seen by a medical professional. The reasons affecting older adult's access to health services are linked with the inadequacy of health care facilities to meet the health needs of older patients. Much of the focus of health services is on children under the age of 5 and mothers. Specialist geriatric care services for diseases common in old age such as Alzheimer's disease or related dementias are fairly limited. There are few specialised geriatric services available in the country. Health care services are available for free in public health facilities but older people face a number of obstacles including a shortage of essential medications, limited access to assistive devices, and perceived negative attitudes, as well as a lack of thoroughness and information sharing from health professionals that attend to them (Joubert & Bradshaw, 2006). All these factors may result in older people experiencing challenges in obtaining appropriate care and support and may also explain their under-utilisation of healthcare services.

Elder abuse occurs when older people are deliberately targeted based on their age and perceived fragility, and a relationship of trust is intentionally established to deceive, exploit, and abuse them (Jacobs, 2023). However, while elder abuse is recognised as a major problem, a review of the literature suggests that it is poorly researched which is surprising given the high levels of crime in South Africa. When compared to other countries, South Africa is known for its high level of crime. It has the third highest crime rate globally, 75.5 cases per 100,000, making it one of the most dangerous and violent countries in the world (World Population Review, 2024). It is also difficult to estimate the magnitude of elder abuse because of under-reporting. A study conducted in the North West province by Bigala and Ayiga (2014) found that elder abuse is prevalent and includes physical, financial, emotional, and sexual abuse. Men were more likely than women to encounter physical violence, but only women reported sexual abuse. Elder abuse negatively impacts quality of life and dignity as the experience is often embarrassing and humiliating especially in the case of sexual abuse (Mtiya-Thimla & Van der Merwe, 2021). It is not uncommon for victims of sexual abuse to feel shame and feelings of stigmatisation.

In South Africa, the belief in witchcraft is very strong, particularly in rural areas. Most often, women are the target of these accusations and they may face mob justice which includes extrajudicial killings, forced exile, and disappearance as well as brutality such as burning, hanging, stoning, and beatings that often result in death (Kay, 2012). Sometimes older people with dementia display symptoms such as confusion, memory loss, and mood alterations which have also resulted in them being labelled as 'bewitched' or 'cursed' (Khonje et al., 2015), making them vulnerable to abuse. The rise in drug and alcohol abuse in communities has also had a significant impact on the elderly. Addicts who are under the influence of substances frequently use aggression against older individuals. Older adults are viewed as vulnerable, their possessions are seized, and their grants taken to support addictions (Kay, 2012). Abuse is typically perpetrated by family members in their own homes, which means many older people do not feel safe in their homes.

As people age, they are less likely to be in formal employment. A number of studies suggest that employment rates decline even before people reach retirement age (Riumallo-Herl et al., 2019). There are lower levels of labour force participation after age 45 years, indicating that a large percentage of the economically active are either not employed or not economically active (Roux & Viljoen, 2018). There have been a number of explanations for this trend. South Africa has one of the highest unemployment rates in the world, with an official unemployment rate of 32.9% in 2024 (Statistics South Africa, 2024). It is therefore a serious concern and older people, like the youth, may battle to secure employment. It is also plausible that older people do not participate in the labour force because of ill-health. They are more likely to suffer from age-related chronic conditions which limits their economic participation in the labour force. Many older adults therefore struggle with financial insecurity due to limited pensions, lack of savings, and limited employment opportunities.

For the majority of older people, the state-sponsored means-tested old age grant is the primary source of income. The old age grant was introduced in the late 1920s but only much later in the early 1990s was access to the grant extended to Black Africans (Ralston et al., 2016). Historically, men aged 65 years of age or older and women aged 60 years or older were eligible for the old age grant. But by 2012, both older men and women qualified for the Older Person's Grant at the age of 60 years. To be eligible men and women had to be aged 60 years and over, they had to have a South African identification document (either citizens, or permanent residents), and they had to comply with the means-test. In 2024, individuals over 60 years receive R2 180 per month, while those aged 75 and above receive approximately R2 200 per month. Numerous studies suggest that the old age grant provides a number of protective benefits for the individual and the household (Ralston et al., 2022; Van Dijk & Mokgala, 2014).

Men and women aged 60 years and older may not be working but this does not mean that they are a financial burden to their families. This is largely because of the means-tested state-supported old age pension system. In the context of high unemployment, the old age pension is critical for the survival of not only the older person but also the household. Numerous studies highlight the protective benefits of pensions for all household members (Ralston et al., 2016; Rossouw, 2017). Most poor households do not have savings because they tend to spend whatever income they have on food. Thus, social grants may constitute their only source of income which provides support to the entire family, without which they will be destitute especially if payments are not made in a timely fashion (Rossouw, 2017). A study by Lloyd-Sherlock et al. (2018) suggests that family members tend to move in with older members who are receiving a pension. Older South Africans (especially Black individuals) feel a moral obligation to share their pensions with family members (Lloyd-Sherlock et al., 2018).

In traditional African societies, old age was viewed as a blessing, and older people were assigned a high status in the community. Older people have traditionally been highly valued members of society. They were the 'transmitters of culture', 'custodians of the secrets of life', or 'the wise ones' (Michel et al., 2019). In addition, they were widely relied on for mediating of family conflicts and the maintenance of peace in the family. They were well-respected and recognised for their knowledge and experience. Over the past few decades, there has been a remarkable shift in attitudes towards older people. Increasing studies suggest that many older people feel that that they are no longer treated with respect and their position has been severely undermined (Michel et al., 2019; Kelly et al., 2019). Today older people are no longer seen as having a role to play in the socialisation and disciplining of young people. In fact, many older people complain that they are no longer given respect by the youth and they feel that there is no reverence for their accumulated knowledge, experience, and authority (Rwezaura, 1989).

Increased longevity is associated with a greater demand for health care. However, the health system is under enormous stress and plagued with a number of challenges including shortage of healthcare workers, poor leadership, and inefficient resource allocation (Kelly et al., 2019). This is despite major strides that have been made in recent years to improve the accessibility and quality of health services. Numerous studies suggest that people of all ages encounter obstacles to effective care in South Africa's public health system, which is also likely to influence how older people perceive public health care (Ameh et al., 2014; Kelly et al., 2019). Older people with lower levels of functional ability experience challenges with transportation to and from healthcare facilities (Phaswana-Mafuya et al., 2013). Moreover, lengthy waiting times at healthcare facilities tend to put extra physical burden on older people. There is also a general shortage of workers equipped with the expertise in managing geriatric issues and chronic diseases experienced by the elderly in South Africa (Phaswana-Mafuya et al., 2013). Care provision to the elderly might lessen their exposure to dire health complications, hence the emphasis on care provision for them is crucial.

As stated by Harandi et al. (2017), care provision is likely the single most influential factor in elderly people's well-being since it not only gives them the tools they need to deal with ageing life challenges but also has a positive impact on both their physical and mental health especially when they receive appropriate care and support. Most often, older people look to other family members for assistance. In the absence of affordable formal care systems outside of the health sector, families are a valuable source of support and care of children, the sick, and the elderly (Apt, 2012). In addition, there are limited affordable retirement or old age homes, which provide an alternative form of housing for the elderly. Traditionally, the expectation has been that the care and support of older people should come from adult children and grandchildren (Nyirenda et al., 2015). However, over time traditional family structures has weakened as a result of younger members migrating to cities and other provinces in search of job opportunities as well as other factors.

Older people are also a valuable source of support for their family members. This may take various forms including material, physical, and emotional support. Often adults who become sick rely on their parents for assistance when they are no longer able to manage by themselves. A number of older adult family members including grandmothers and aunts, but also grandfathers and uncles, frequently play a role in meeting the diverse needs of children. Older women, in particular, have been a critical resource in the fight against HIV/AIDS and lessening its effects throughout sub-Saharan Africa. They assumed the majority of the massive additional burdens that the HIV/AIDS epidemic have placed on families and society. Also, when their children migrated for the purposes of work, grandmothers took responsibility for the care of their grandchildren. In such situations, the old age grant was invaluable in providing them with the financial resources to attend to the needs of the orphaned children under their care. The informal caregiving that is provided by older people often occurs in the context of high levels of poverty, and inequality, inadequate support, as well as a number of the other challenges frequently facing them.

Summary and Organisation of the Volume

In South Africa the older population has been steadily increasing as more people are living longer than ever before. Older people constitute a significant share of the total population of South Africa but their situation is rarely well-understood. This book argues that an ageing population is likely to have major implications for the country, not least as a major driver of the growth of the population but also increasing demands on resources and services. However, an ageing population also brings greater opportunities as older people are often a valuable source of support and care in many households. This book acknowledges the importance of research on the situation of older people, while taking into account the need for greater planning around the growing number of older people in the country. This volume is organised into two parts. The first part sets the scene for the volume, profiling the situation of older people in South Africa. The second part examines case studies drawing on qualitative and quantitative data to better illuminate the social realities of ageing in the country.

The Constitution of the Republic of South African includes a Bill of Human Rights that protects the rights of all citizens and forbids discrimination based on age. In 1994, the first democratically elected government pledged to rebuild and develop the country and its people, despite a legacy of injustice and human rights violations caused by colonialism and apartheid (Lombard & Kruger, 2009). The Older Persons Act, 2006, was introduced to deal effectively with the situation of people aged 60 years and older and advance the plight of older people. The intention of this

Act is "to protect, promote and maintain the status, well-being and security of older persons". The emphasis on older persons is in line with the 2030 United Nations Agenda for Sustainable Development. Through this, the international community has set itself the target to better the lives of the most vulnerable and marginalised including older people.

The challenges posed by the rising numbers of older persons in South Africa require urgent attention because of widespread poverty, unemployment, inadequate health systems, poorly managed institutions, and the heavy burden of communicable and non-communicable diseases facing the country. It is therefore imperative that there is adequate planning for the ageing population. This is in line with the 2030 Agenda for Sustainable Development which outlines a plan of action for achieving sustainable development while also realising the human rights of all people, particularly the most vulnerable including older people. This book acknowledges the shared vision of the 2030 Agenda by exploring the experiences of older people who are often in the margins of society. Older people are key to attaining the Sustainable Development Goals whose primary goal is to *"leave no one behind"*. This is best attained through delving into new and emerging insights in a country like South Africa that is undergoing rapid change and transformation.

References

Aboderin, I. A., & Gelfand, L. (2019). *A demographic dividend for Africa: The value of investing in the older population*. African Population and Health Research Centre.

Ameh, S., Gómez-Olivé, F. X., Kahn, K., Tollman, S. M., & Klipstein-Grobusch, K. (2014). Predictors of health care use by adults 50 years and over in a rural South African setting. *Global Health Action, 7*, 24771.

Apt, N. A. (2012). Aging in Africa: Past experiences and strategic directions. *Ageing International, 37*(1), 93–103.

Baloyi, M. E. (2015). A pastoral investigation into some of the challenges associated with aging and retirement in the South African context. *In die Skriflig, 49*(3), 1–10.

Bigala, P., & Ayiga, N. (2014). Prevalence and predictors of elder abuse in Mafikeng Local Municipality in South Africa. *African Population Studies, 28*(1), 463–474.

Chigali, G. M., Marais, M., & Mpofu, R. M. B. (2002). An investigative study of the experiences of elderly people in a South African Black Township. *South African Journal of Physiotherapy, 58*(3), 21–26.

Gaskin, C. J., & Orellana, L. (2018). Factors associated with physical activity and sedentary behavior in older adults from six low-and middle-income countries. *International Journal of Environmental Research and Public Health, 15*(5), 908.

Harandi, T. F., Taghinasab, M. M., & Nayeri, T. D. (2017). The correlation of social support with mental health: A meta-analysis. *Electronic Physician, 9*(9), 5212–5222.

Jacobs, R. (2023). *Elder abuse in South Africa: Measurement, prevalence and risk.* Unpublished doctoral dissertation, University of Cape Town.

Joubert, J., & Bradshaw, D. (2006). Population ageing and health challenges. In K. Steyn, J. Fourie, & N. Temple (Eds.), *Chronic diseases of lifestyle in South Africa* (pp. 1995–2005). South African Medical Research Council.

Kay, R. (2012). *Older persons in South Africa: The forgotten victims.* South African Older Persons' Forum.

Kelly, G., Mrengqwa, L., & Geffen, L. (2019). "They don't care about us": Older people's experiences of primary healthcare in Cape Town, South Africa. *BMC Geriatrics, 19*(1), 1–14.

Khonje, V., Milligan, C., Yako, Y., Mabelane, M., Borochowitz, K. E., & De Jager, C. A. (2015). Knowledge, attitudes and beliefs about dementia in an urban Xhosa-speaking community in South Africa. *Advances in Alzheimer's Disease, 4*(2), 21–36.

Lloyd-Sherlock, P., Penhale, B., & Ayiga, N. (2018). Financial abuse of older people in low and middle-income countries: The case of South Africa. *Journal of Elder Abuse & Neglect, 30*(3), 236–246.

Lombard, A., & Kruger, E. (2009). Older persons: The case of South Africa. *Ageing International, 34*, 119–135.

Mfene, X. P., & Pillay, B. J. (2023). Knowledge of dementia and dementia care in a cross-sectional sample of individuals living in rural and urban areas in KwaZulu-Natal, South Africa. *South Africa Journal of Psychology, 53*(2), 265–274.

Michel, J., Stuckelberger, A., Tediosi, F., Evans, D. & van Eeuwijk. (2019). The roles of a Grandmother in African societies – please do not send them to old people's homes. *Journal of Global Health, 9*(1), 010306.

Mtiya-Thimla, G., & Van der Merwe, M. (2021). The experiences of abused older persons in resource-poor settings. *Social Work, 57*(2), 226–243.

Mussie, K. M., Setchell, J., Elger, B. S., Kaba, M., Memirie, S. T., & Wangmo, T. (2022). Care of older persons in Eastern Africa: A scoping review of ethical issues. *Frontiers in Public Health, 10*, 923097.

National Institute for Communicable Diseases (NICD). (2020). *Clinical management of suspected or confirmed Covid-19 disease*. NICD.

Ngubane, M. Z., Mndebele, S., & Kaseeram, I. (2023). Economic growth, unemployment and poverty: Linear and non-linear evidence from South Africa. *Heliyon, 9*(10), e20267.

Ntozini, A., & Abdullahi, A. A. (2021). Loneliness and psychological well-being among the elderly in Buffalo City, South Africa. *Journal of Psychology in Africa, 31*(4), 383–389.

Nyirenda, M., Evandrou, M., Mutevedzi, P., Hosegood, V., Falkingham, J., & Newell, M. L. (2015). Who cares? Implications of care-giving and-receiving by HIV-infected or-affected older people on functional disability and emotional wellbeing. *Ageing & Society, 35*(1), 169–202.

Padayachey, U., Ramlall, S., & Chipps, J. (2017). Depression in older adults: Prevalence and risk factors in a primary health care sample. *South African Family Practice, 59*(2), 61–66.

Peltzer, K., & Phaswana-Mafuya, N. (2013). Depression and associated factors in older adults in South Africa. *Global Health Action, 6*(1), 18871.

Phaswana-Mafuya, N., Peltzer, K., Chirinda, W., Kose, Z., Hoosain, E., Ramlagan, S., Tabane, C., & Davids, A. (2013). Self-rated health and associated factors among older South Africans: Evidence from the study on global ageing and adult health. *Global Health Action, 6*(1), 19880.

Ralston, M., Schatz, E., Menken, J., Gómez-Olivé, F. X., & Tollman, S. (2016). Who benefits—Or does not—From South Africa's old age pension? Evidence from characteristics of rural pensioners and non-pensioners. *International Journal of Environmental Research and Public Health, 13*(2), 85.

Ralston, M., Jennings, E., & Schatz, E. (2022). Who is at risk? Social support, relationship dissolution, and illness in a rural context. *Sociological Inquiry, 92*(3), 1053–1082.

Riumallo-Herl, C., Canning, D., & Kabudula, C. (2019). Health inequalities in the South African elderly: The importance of the measure of social-economic status. *The Journal of the Economics of Ageing, 14*, 100191.

Roebuck, J. (1979). When does old age begin? The evolution of the English definition. *Journal of Social History, 12*(3), 416–428.

Rossouw, J. (2017). Why social grants matter in South Africa: They support 33% of the nation. *The Conversation*, 16 February.

Roux, A., & Viljoen, D. (2018). Using futures studies methodologies to explore the economic participation of the older cohorts of South Africa's population towards 2030. *Journal of Futures Studies, 23*(1), 5–22.

Rwezaura, B. A. (1989). Changing community obligations to the elderly in contemporary Africa. *Journal of Social Development in Africa, 4*(1), 5–24.

Schatz, E., Seeley, J., Negin, J., & Mugisha, J. (2018). They 'don't cure old age': Older Ugandans' delays to health-care access. *Ageing & Society, 38*(11), 2197–2217.

Solanki, G., Kelly, G., Cornell, J., Daviaud, E., & Geffen, L. (2019). Population ageing in South Africa: Trends, impact, and challenges for the health sector. In *South African health review 2019*. Health Systems Trust.

Statistics South Africa. (2011). *Census 2011: Profile of older persons in South Africa*. Statistics South Africa.

Statistics South Africa. (2019). *Mid-year population estimates, 2019*. Statistics South Africa.

Statistics South Africa. (2022). *Mid-year population estimates, 2022*. Statistics South Africa.

Statistics South Africa. (2023). *The social profile of older persons, 2017–2021*. Statistics South Africa.

Statistics South Africa. (2024). *Quarterly Labour Force Survey (QLFS), Quarter 1: 2024*. Statistics South Africa.

Tomlinson, M., Grimsrud, A. T., Stein, D. J., Williams, D. R., & Myer, L. (2009). The epidemiology of major depression in South Africa: Results from the South African Stress and Health study: Mental health. *South African Medical Journal, 99*(5), 368–373.

United Nations. (2022). *South Africa National Human Development Report 2022*. United Nations.

Van Dijk, H. G., & Mokgala, M. (2014). Does the administration of the Old Age Grant really benefit the rural poor? *African Journal of Public Affairs, 7*(4), 82–96.

Walsh, K., Scharf, T., & Keating, N. (2017). Social exclusion of older persons: A scoping review and conceptual framework. *European Journal of Ageing, 14*(1), 81–98.

World Health Organization (WHO). (2019). *Risk reduction of cognitive decline and dementia: WHO guidelines*. World Health Organization.

World Population Review. (2024). *Crime rate by country 2024*. https://worldpopulationreview.com/country-rankings/crime-rate-by-country

Yaya, S., Idriss-Wheeler, D., Sanogo, N. A., Vezina, M., & Bishwajit, G. (2020). Self- reported activities of daily living, health and quality of life among older adults in South Africa and Uganda: A cross sectional study. *BMC Geriatrics, 20*, 402.

2

Ageing in South Africa: Trends and Determinants

Sachin Sewpersad and Pranitha Maharaj

Abstract South Africa is undergoing major demographic changes with a significant proportion of the population aged 60 years and over. This chapter provides an in-depth examination of population ageing in South Africa, with a specific focus on the pace, magnitude, and determinants. An ageing population is largely driven by decreases in fertility and mortality. While more South Africans are living longer, this does not mean that they are living in good health due to health issues and functional limitations that accompany ageing. The ageing population exhibits differences in relation to age, gender, and other characteristics, including living arrangements, marital status, and use of healthcare resources. As population ageing is increasingly highlighted as a concern, projections and forecasting will allow for effective implementation of initiatives at varying levels. This chapter highlights the urgent need for infrastructure

S. Sewpersad (✉) • P. Maharaj
School of Built Environment and Development Studies, University of KwaZulu-Natal, Durban, South Africa
e-mail: SewpersadS@ukzn.ac.za; maharajp7@ukzn.ac.za

P. Maharaj (ed.), *Navigating Ageing in South Africa*, Sustainable Development Goals Series, https://doi.org/10.1007/978-981-97-9088-3_2

and services to be accessible and available to accommodate the ageing population.

Keywords Older people • Ageing populations • Age structure • Determinants • South Africa

Introduction

South Africa is undergoing major, rapid demographic changes and even though much of the country's population is relatively youthful, a significant proportion of the population is aged 60 years and older. In the past, a relatively small percentage of the population was aged 60 years and older; however, this has been rapidly changing. As life expectancy increases and more people are living past age 60, there is a higher chronic disease burden and increased demand on the health system. Moreover, there is an increase in the need for social grants, pension benefits, and other publicly funded programmes. However, the country's current older population is continuously marginalised against broader efforts to achieve economic and social development. With the majority of the population aged below 45 years, most development strategies within the country focus on maximising the potential of the demographic dividend (Roux & Viljoen, 2018). This chapter starts by providing a profile of older people in South Africa, with a specific focus on the pace, magnitude, and determinants of population ageing within the country.

Population Ageing in South Africa

At present, the population of South Africa is approximately 62 million. Older people have historically constituted a small proportion of South Africa's population when compared to any other age group. However, as fertility levels continuously falls and life expectancy continues to rise, the older population is expected to expand and live longer (He et al., 2020). South Africa's life expectancy has increased over the past few decades. This is largely due to increased access to HIV antiretroviral treatment, improvements in public health interventions, as well as advancements in sanitation, housing, and nutrition (Aboyade et al., 2016). While life expectancy dropped slightly as a result of the global COVID-19 pandemic, it later experienced an improvement as vaccines were developed and health interventions and treatment for infections improved.

The population aged 60 and older is growing at a rate of about 2.11% per year (Statistics South Africa, 2022c), and over the next few decades a further increase is certain due to increased life expectancy and a lower mortality rate. Between 2002 and 2022, South Africa's elderly population was estimated to increase from 3.3 million to 5.7 million, with a 69.7% increase over this period (Solanki et al., 2019). The growth rate of older South Africans rose from 1.08% for the period 2002–2003 to 2.88% for the period 2019–2020 (Statistics South Africa, 2022c). However, given the levels of mortality among older people during the COVID-19 pandemic, the growth rate among the elderly had drastically declined from 2.88% for the period 2019–2020 to 1.47% for the period 2020–2021. However, this increased back to 2.11% in the period 2021–2022 due to early interventions to curb the further spread of the coronavirus (Statistics South Africa, 2022c).

In 2022, South Africa's population aged 60 years and older was estimated at more than 5.5 million, representing a 9.2% share of the total population (Statistics South Africa, 2023a). Between 2017 and 2022, the older population increased by 12.3%, with all provinces recording an increase in the percentage of older persons during this period (Statistics South Africa, 2023a). However, trends in ageing have shown that two provinces—Gauteng and Western Cape—will experience the largest growth of its ageing population over the upcoming decades. Projections suggests that rapid ageing will continue to occur in South Africa and by 2050, out of a projected population of 75.5 million, the percentage of people aged 60 years and older will be around 16%, or approximately 12 million people (Statistics South Africa, 2019). An increasing older population has major and long-term implications for future development in the country.

Key Drivers of Population Ageing

Before examining the characteristics of population ageing, it is important to understand the demographic determinants. The age structure of the population is dependent on the interplay of three main dynamics, namely, fertility, mortality, and migration. However, fertility and mortality are far more significant demographic factors contributing to the increase in the ageing population than migration as people seldom migrate at older ages (He et al., 2020). Although the migratory movements of people in and out of a population does substantially impact the age structure, it is the demographic phenomenon of decreasing fertility and mortality that makes the largest contribution to an ageing population (He et al., 2020). The effect of decreasing fertility rates in South Africa, coupled with decreasing mortality, will inevitably result in an older population in the future.

A greater life expectancy in the population is indicative of improvements and developments in health and a decline in mortality (Rademeyer & Maharaj, 2020). Over the past few years, life expectancy increased dramatically. While life expectancy determines the number of years a person is expected to live based on the statistical average, a healthy life expectancy measures the number of years an individual is expected to live in good health, based on both period life expectancy and a measure of self-rated health (WHO, 2020). An analysis of life expectancy and healthy life expectancy data highlights that while life expectancy in 2019 was an average of 65.3 years at birth, healthy life expectancy was only 56.2 years (WHO, 2020). This suggests that, on average, approximately 9 years of elderly life are spent in poor health.

Women constitute a significantly larger proportion of the older population, as their life expectancy is greater than that of men, with the female share increasing with age. Mortality rates of women are lower than men at older ages; therefore, the proportion of women in the older population grows substantially with advancing age. In 2001, 7.3% of the South African population was 60 years and over, and this is projected to increase to 24% by the year 2050 (WHO, 2015). In other words, almost a quarter of the South African population is projected to be aged 60 years and over.

The increase in the ageing population is due to the large proportion of the working-age population who will in the future contribute to the ageing population.

The other demographic dynamic that contributes to an ageing population is the decline in fertility. Over the last several decades, fertility levels have been steadily declining in many countries globally, though at a much slower pace in Africa. While the population of Africa is projected to increase dramatically over the next few years, South Africa's fertility levels have been declining. South Africa is one of the first countries in sub-Saharan Africa to experience an overall fertility decline (Palamuleni et al., 2007). The overall fertility rate has fallen steadily over time, from 6.0 in the mid-1950s to about 4.3 in the 1980s (Caldwell & Caldwell, 1993; DoH, 1998). In 2021, the fertility rate for South Africa was 2.3 births per woman, a 0.89% decline from 2020 (United Nations, 2022). As of 2024, fertility rates are estimated at 2.2 births per woman, a 0.78% decline from 2023 (United Nations, 2022). It has also been speculated that the country's fertility rates could possibly drop to replacement levels (Swartz, 2009). However, a certain degree of variation in fertility levels exists across geographical areas and racial groups.

The fertility rate of Whites is relatively low and is reaching replacement level—a trend observed in more developed countries. This decline among Whites occurred at a much earlier stage than for the other racial groups. The fertility rate of Africans has also been declining but the pace has only increased in the last four decades. The decline in the fertility rate of Africans has been more rapid in the urban than rural areas (Palamuleni et al., 2007). Despite this, the fertility rate in South Africa is much lower than those recorded elsewhere in sub-Saharan Africa, where the overall total fertility rates are approximately 5 children per woman (Tesfa et al., 2023). The current fertility rate of 2.2 is expected to decline further. This trend is likely to have major implications for the workforce, leading to a sharp fall in the number of young people entering the labour market over time. As a result, in the next few decades, the supply of older workers relative to the supply of new workers will rise sharply.

The ageing population of South Africa will continue growing for several decades. The increasing number of older people in the country is a demographic phenomenon linked to decreases in both fertility and mortality, and is not merely a result of economic progress. While these demographic trends are inevitable, it urgently calls for prompt and applicable policy interventions and development initiatives to cater for the needs of the future demographic composition of the country.

Age-Sex Differentials

With a growing older population, the country's age-sex structure begins to lose its characteristic pyramid-like shape and turns into one that is more uniform, as the population of youth declines. The age structure of the South African population has been changing over time, with the majority being relatively more youthful and of working ages, keeping the dependency ratio of the country relatively stable for now but this will soon change. In 2023, the population of working age women in South Africa reached almost 20.7 million, while the number of working age men reached roughly 20.4 million (Statistics South Africa, 2023b). This is not surprising, since it is widely recognised that the South African population is youthful. However, the country will face a substantially diminished working-age population. While the working age population constitutes the majority in South Africa now, it is important to note that this demographic will also continue to age over time. Compounded with declining fertility rates, these projections suggest that social and economic support for the country's ageing population may not be sufficient in the future as there will be a greater ratio of older population to working age population. The increase in the dependency ratio will have negative implications for the South African ageing population, especially if the increase continues in the years beyond 2050.

Another important variable to consider when analysing data on the ageing population is gender. Gathering data on gender differentials is vital, as the continuation of gender-based inequality serves as a hindrance to South Africa's growth (Dalu et al., 2020). In South Africa, between 2017 and 2022, the sex ratio of older people declined slightly (from 65 men per 100 women in 2017 to 64 men per 100 women in 2022), indicating that the proportion of women in the older population had increased over time (Statistics South Africa, 2022a, 2023a). These trends are starkly visible when analysing the age-sex structure of the country's population over time. Thus, in South Africa there are more women aged 60 years and older than men. This also applies to the oldest age groups who are 80 years and above, with 68 men for every 100 women, or in other words, slightly more women (25%) than men. This is expected, given that most studies suggest that women live longer than men, and thus they form the majority in the oldest category. It is important to ascertain whether policies are attuned to the predominantly ageing female population. The feminisation of the older population has the potential of becoming one of the biggest challenges of gender equality. This is because life expectancy is generally higher for women, many of whom struggle to meet their basic needs and suffer significant health inequities, poor financial security, and inadequate standards of living at older ages (Rademeyer & Maharaj, 2020).

Marital status

Marriage is a vital source of social support for older people, serving as a safety net and allowing them to better cope with physical decline and poor health as they age (Freedman et al., 2019). Marriage has protective benefits for the couple as it can provide them with social and material support. Furthermore, married individuals are usually healthier and live longer lives than those who are not married (Lawrence et al., 2019). Analysing marriage statistics provides a good indication of the socio-economic status of households, and since married individuals have better health than non-married individuals, it serves as an indicator of a population's health status (Waite, 2004). In South Africa, the largest share of older people is married legally, followed by those who are widowed. However, between 2017 and 2021, there was a drop in the number of legally married older people while those who were widowed increased (Statistics South Africa, 2018, 2022b).

Looking at gender differentials, older men are more likely to be married than older women. The number of men that were legally married and living with their partners surpassed that of women for both 2017 and 2021 (Statistics South Africa, 2018, 2022b). Men also tend to experience greater health benefits from marriage than women, possibly because they receive more emotional support and are encouraged to adopt more healthy behaviours, typically from their wives (Carr & Springer, 2010). There is also evidence to demonstrate that unmarried women have higher psychological well-being than unmarried men (Hsu & Barrett, 2020).

As most of them are married, older men are in an advantaged position; by being married, they enjoy better health and a better socio-economic position than the older men who are not married. With women, the majority are disadvantaged in terms of marital status, as fewer (32%) are married or in a consensual union (Statistics South Africa, 2022b). This means that almost 70% of older South African women have a decreased health and socio-economic status in comparison to older women who are married or in a consensual union. In addition, marital dissolution is associated with poorer mental health in South Africa, where marital breakdown and spousal death is prevalent (Jennings et al., 2022).

Changes in marital rates have also had significant effects on household formation as marriage is closely related to women's economic welfare in a way that is not quite the same for men (Thornton, 2023). Historically, the female disadvantage in the labour market and involvement in household activities meant that women were dependent on men's earnings, often via marriage. However, as male unemployment increased towards the end of apartheid, marital rates consistently declined as the incentive for women to marry had greatly fallen (Thornton, 2023).

Living Arrangements

The living arrangements of older people are determined by many social and economic factors. These factors include relationship with family members, marital status, financial well-being, health status, and family size. Furthermore, family structure, kinship patterns, as well as cultural traditions also play a role in influencing patterns of living arrangements among older people (Lombard & Kruger, 2009; Velkoff, 2001). Living arrangements form a critical aspect of older people's lives because how they live and who they live with undoubtedly affect their daily life, health, and well-being (De Jong Gierveld et al., 2000).

While the living environment of older adults plays an important role in their well-being, it also influences their quality of life and physical activity level. Older people who live in community or family settings tend to have a higher quality of life and physical activity levels than those who live in institutions such as old age homes. This is attributed to the physical and physiological benefits of physical activity such as regular exercise and household activities (Ramocha et al., 2017). As a result, independence and mental health among older persons are improved leading to an overall improved quality of life (Ramocha et al., 2017). Disability also plays a major role in the needs of older people and their ability to provide support to others in the household. The roles and expectations of household members fluctuate depending on the care and resources members provide or that they need, resulting in some members receiving more than they give, and others giving more than they receive (Schatz et al., 2018).

South Africa's older population is largely income poor, and living in large, multi-generational, female-dominated, and female-headed households (Lombard & Kruger 2009). Ageing-in-place along with poor alternatives to family-based care means that multi-generational living arrangements (residences that typically have more than one adult generation of family members) continue to be the dominant living arrangement for older people in much of sub-Saharan Africa (Schatz et al., 2018). This is particularly the case for rural South Africa, where the living situations of older persons have been affected by high levels of mortality in the middle generation due to HIV as well as the migration of young adults (Hosegood, 2009). In addition, older people may also provide additional care for other members of the household, including the sick, and often incur extra costs to meet the requirements of the family (Alexio et al., 2019). Although South Africa has no housing policy for older people, the Ministry of Social Development encourages older individuals to remain living with family and therefore age-in-place for as long as possible; further postulating that family has the primary responsibility to care for and shelter elderly relatives (Ferreira, 2010). The government is overwhelmed by the demand for social housing by adults of all ages, claiming lack of resources (Ferreira, 2010).

Multi-generational living arrangements also benefit older people, whose family acts as a source of caregiving. Caregiving may include assisting older people with one or more activities important for daily living such as bathing and dressing, paying bills, shopping, safety features, medical care, socialisation, chores, errands, finances, and providing transportation (Schulz, 2006). It also may involve emotional support and help with managing a chronic disease or disability. This is known as in-home care, which is provided by a relative or kin and is considered to be the best to meet the well-being of the person receiving the care (Brear et al., 2024). Older persons also make financial and caregiving contributions to households, and this may be necessary in some living arrangements (Schatz et al., 2018). In this sense, older persons may be considered productive where there are higher expectations and needs, and they are contributing emotional and physical labour for themselves and others (Schatz et al., 2018).

Residential or assisted living care facilities are commonly accessed by older people, depending on functional need or social indigence (Ferreira, 2010). Private old age homes are usually available for the few who can afford the monthly fees (Nzima & Maharaj, 2020). Often, it is mainly older Whites living in these private old age homes (Lloyd-Sherlock et al., 2018). There are striking variations in intergenerational households by race. Older Whites were most likely to live in single-generation households in contrast to older Indians, who were more likely to reside in second-generation households. Multi-generation households were more common among older Black Africans and Coloureds than other groups. Generally older Black Africans prefer to co-reside with family where possible and share their pension income within the household (Mtshali, 2016). Only a small number of older Whites receive a social pension and prefer living independently if they are functionally and financially able to do so (Ferreira, 2010).

Education and Technology

Literacy is an important indicator of well-being of older people and their involvement in society. For older people, literacy and education has significant benefits that offers socialisation, mental stimulation, and allowing them to stay updated with new information. Education also prevents social exclusion and isolation, as social interaction is facilitated by various forms of communication technology. This is increasingly instrumental in enabling older people to overcome social isolation and loneliness, allowing them to maintain close contact with family and friends (Grey et al., 2024). Literacy also benefits older people by allowing them to engage in various media platforms to keep up with current affairs and engage in social matters. Moreover, low health literacy can promote healthcare and self-management of disease (Geboers et al., 2018). However, older adults with poor cognitive functioning and high levels of cognitive decline are at risk for low health literacy.

Functional literacy includes an individual's capacity to engage in all activities that is required to function effectively in society (UNESCO, 2021). The functional literacy rates of older South African men increased from almost 63% in 2017 to almost 70% in 2021, while older women experienced an increase in literacy rates from approximately 55% in 2017 to slightly over 60% in 2021 (Statistics South Africa, 2023a). For both years, older men were more likely than older women to be functionally literate. There are also disparities in literacy rates between the various racial groups with older Black Africans lagging behind all other groups. On the other hand, older Whites were universally functionally literate (Statistics South Africa, 2023a).

Level of education was relatively high among older people. In South Africa, for both 2017 and 2021, older men and women had obtained some secondary schooling as the highest level of education. However, older men's educational attainment tends to be higher than that of older women, especially for completed secondary and higher education levels. In contrast, the educational attainment of older women tends to be higher than that of older men at lower levels of education, including those with no schooling and primary levels in both 2017 and 2021 (Statistics South Africa, 2023a).

Over the last several years, the world has become more technologically advanced with an increase in the use of digital platforms even among older people. This is especially because it is an easy means to connect to others and evade loneliness. Digital technology is also becoming increasingly important for functional independence for older people (Czaja, 2016). The prevalence of internet connections among South Africa's various racial groups displayed a consistent pattern between 2017 and 2019, with a higher percentage of older Whites having access to the internet, while older Black Africans had lower internet access. In 2019, approximately 45% of older Whites had internet access in comparison to 1.5% of older Black Africans (Statistics South Africa, 2023a).

Economic Activities and Income

A rapidly ageing population contains fewer working-age individuals and therefore risks a shortage of qualified workers in the economy, making it more difficult for businesses to fill in-demand roles (Borji, 2013). An economy that cannot fill in-demand occupations faces adverse consequences such as declining productivity, higher labour costs, delayed business expansion, and reduced international competitiveness. In some instances, a supply shortage may push up wages, thereby causing wage inflation and creating a vicious cycle of price/wage spiral (Borji, 2013). However, as people are living longer, they are also becoming more productive at older ages. There is evidence to suggest that the health status of older people has improved dramatically over the past several decades (National Academies of Sciences, Engineering, and Medicine, 2022; Statistics South Africa, 2023a). This improvement in health has also coincided with a sharp decline in physical job demands and, with the increasing digitisation of the workforce, this trend is expected to continue (Solem et al., 2023).

Workplace culture, such as prejudice and discrimination, and retirement financial incentives often discourage work at older ages. However, emerging evidence now suggests that retirement at a pre-determined age is not necessarily a natural step in modern work life (OECD, 2020). The enhanced ability to work at older ages has become increasingly common alongside the improved health that accompanies a longer life expectancy (National Academies of Sciences, Engineering, and Medicine, 2022). The majority of older people in South Africa has never enjoyed access to employment in the formal sector owing to past discriminatory practices, so they do not enjoy secure retirement benefits (Lombard & Kruger, 2009). Furthermore, South Africa currently has a high unemployment rate of approximately 32.1% (Statistics South Africa, 2024). This is due to a combination of structural shortcomings such as a lack of skills, limited access to quality education and training, and inadequate job creation. This has ultimately culminated in a large portion of the population unable to find gainful employment, which also affects older people. Being out of the labour force is directly linked to lower incomes and thus lower capacity to consume.

While the challenges presented by an ageing workforce are different for developing countries, as people age, they are less likely to work because of ill health. Many of the underlying factors associated with the decision to retire are similar and the implications of an ageing workforce for firms are comparable across more developed and developing countries. Demographic trends and the economic, social, and health-related factors that impact on the decision to retire have, therefore, become critical points of analysis in the context of a recognised need to encourage workers to remain in their jobs for longer. This need together with a growing body of research directed towards retirement trends in developed countries assist in identifying the challenges presented by an ageing workforce in developing countries.

With regard to economic activity, men aged 60 and over are more economically active than women (Statistics South Africa, 2023a). Labour force participation by the older population still remains quite high in South Africa. Older people in South Africa may continue to participate in the labour force partly due to difficulties in securing finances in their old age. Employment rates are higher among older people who do not receive a pension, and considering that South Africa has a high economically active older population, this suggests that they are more likely to participate in the labour force in the absence of pension benefits (Tshaka et al., 2023). Continuous engagement in the paid labour force is an important part of maintaining active involvement and development of older persons in society (Statistics South Africa, 2023a).

Social Grants

During the apartheid era, Black South Africans were consistently excluded from most social transfers, and, to a large extent, from public pensions (Tondini et al., 2017). This occurred in several different ways: the means test was set at different levels for different races, and was significantly lower for Black Africans and Coloureds. Moreover, the benefits paid when actually eligible only made up one tenth of the amount paid to Whites (Tondini et al., 2017). However, in the early 1990s, the South African government introduced the old age pension administered by the South African Social Security Agency (SASSA)—a government-based agency. The grants are paid out to all South Africans who meet the qualifying requirements, offering relief to vulnerable older people aged 60 years and older, and serves as a valuable source of income for certain households. The social grants are means-tested and are crucial in cushioning recipients against abject poverty and inequality. The increasing life expectancy for both older men and women necessitates greater social protection for them in the form of old age pensions, health services, and housing (Pillay & Maharaj, 2013).

The gradual erosion of the family support system and the use of their meagre incomes to bring up orphaned grandchildren results in an increasing number of older persons becoming actively involved in the struggle to earn a living (Makiwane & Kwizera, 2006). Extreme poverty and high levels of unemployment in South Africa have resulted in many elderly people being the sole members bringing in an income in a household, thus having to support the entire family with the state pension (Lombard & Kruger, 2009). In South Africa, over 3.8 million persons aged 60 years and older received a social grant in 2021 compared to over 3.1 million in 2017 (Statistics South Africa, 2023a). Approximately two-thirds of older South Africans received social grants in both 2017 and 2021 (Statistics South Africa, 2023a). While the South African old age pension is too small to be an effective means to support their children and grandchildren or to eradicate poverty, it is still regarded as a major source of income to support poor families (Lam et al., 2006).

Social pensions for the elderly in South Africa are widely viewed as a key aspect of the South African government's poverty-alleviation programme (Patel & Triegaardt, 2008). Thus, the state pension in South Africa closes the gap between poor households with access to wage income and those without (Outlioua & Fazouane 2023). In rural areas, combined formal support from social grants offer a form of social protection by creating a web of financial support for family and relatives of older people (Ralston et al., 2022). Although South Africa's social pension system is among the most far-reaching and generous in the developing world, it does not make a significant contribution to the independent living of most elderly people in South Africa (Edmonds et al., 2005). However, it is still regarded as the most effective mechanism for the alleviation of household poverty.

Ageing and Health

Population ageing is often accompanied by changes in the health profile of the population. While increased longevity and improved health among older people represents significant achievements for any country, these trends are not without significant challenges. As life expectancy increases, so does the size of the ageing population as older people start living longer than before. A longer life, however, is not necessarily a healthier life. As people live longer, they are more likely to experience functional limitations. One study found that 38.4% of South Africans between ages 65 and 74 have limitations in daily activities of living such as eating, bathing, dressing, getting in and out of bed, or using the toilet (WHO, 2015). This means that an increasingly larger share of South Africa's population is impacted by limitations in daily living activities and a declining quality of life.

As people age, they are more likely to experience a decline in their health and correspondingly low levels of well-being (Maharaj & Roberts, 2021). It has been established that ageing is a significant risk factor for the development of multiple chronic diseases and infectious diseases. It may be difficult to fully assess the impact of ageing on disease profiles, especially since data on these conditions are not disaggregated by age in the public sector (Solanki et al., 2019). This further makes it difficult to assess the consequences on health services and expenditure in the public sector. There are still health disparities in post-apartheid South Africa by race. A study using a nationally representative sample of South Africans 50 years and older demonstrates how health status differs vastly among older South Africans of different population groups (Peltzer et al., 2019). Black Africans struggle with lower cognitive functioning, while Whites have poor self-reported health status. Coloured older people mainly report poor self-reported health status, lower grip strength, arthritis, hypertension, stroke and/or angina, and low vision, and Indians mainly suffer from poor functional disability, arthritis, and diabetes (Peltzer et al., 2019).

Older people are more likely to experience several degenerative health conditions at the same time. These are often the consequence of multiple underlying factors and include frailty, urinary incontinence, falls, delirium, and pressure ulcers (Inouye et al., 2007). In addition, the emergence of several complex health conditions is common among older people (WHO, 2022). The three health conditions most common among older South Africans are hypertension, diabetes mellitus, and asthma. The prevalence of hypertension increases with age, and is a readily treatable risk factor for the most common causes of morbidity and mortality among older adults (Lloyd-Sherlock et al., 2014). Other common conditions in older age include hearing loss, cataracts and refractive errors, back and neck pain and osteoarthritis, chronic obstructive pulmonary disease, depression, and dementia (WHO, 2022). Between 2017 and 2021, the percentage of older people who suffered from hypertension and asthma decreased, while the number of older people who suffered from diabetes mellitus increased (Statistics South Africa, 2023a). In 2017, it was more likely for older women to suffer from all five listed chronic conditions when compared to older men. In 2021, it was noted that older women were more likely to have diabetes than men (Statistics South Africa, 2023a).

There are also rural–urban health disparities among older people in the country with urban dwellers reporting a higher prevalence of diabetes and better cognitive functioning than rural dwellers (Peltzer et al., 2019). Moreover, functional disability is possibly higher among rural than urban older adults (Peltzer et al., 2019). It is also more likely for older people in rural areas to be underweight than older people in urban areas, while obesity may have a higher prevalence among urban older adults (Peltzer et al., 2019).

The dual burden of HIV and TB are among the most common infectious diseases affecting older adults with an estimated 60% of persons diagnosed with TB being infected with HIV at the same time (van de Water et al., 2023). In the last several years, this risk was compounded by the COVID-19 pandemic, with older people being among the most at risk for infection and mortality caused by the virus. South Africa is among the 30 high-burden tuberculosis (TB) countries and on its own, the country accounts for approximately 3% of cases globally (NDoH, 2018). Older South Africans are not specifically targeted for HIV and TB prevention and testing. Medical providers, especially at the community healthcare level, may fail to suspect or test for infections in the older population cohorts (Akokuwebe et al., 2024). This then results in the diagnosis of diseases among older people being ignored, delayed, or postponed. Approximately 25.9% of older adults with HIV and TB are aged 50–54, the majority of whom are women (Akokuwebe et al., 2024).

The stringent lockdown measures resulted in varied and far-reaching consequences, which adversely affected the health, well-being, and economic situation of older people. While the majority of cases were mild to moderate, those who were more severely affected required intensive hospital care and they felt the health effects of COVID-19 for a longer period of time (Yelin et al., 2020). Thus, COVID-19 infections had created long-term health issues, which are particularly debilitating for older persons (Naidoo et al., 2022). While there is no specific way to treat the disease, vaccines were rapidly developed and administered in different stages. First preference was given to older people due to their excessive vulnerability and increased risk of infection, severe illness, and mortality from the disease (NICD & NDoH, 2022). Older persons were particularly vulnerable to succumbing to COVID-19, with up to 25% of these deaths accounted for by people aged 70–79 years (Calderón-Larrañaga et al., 2020). While old age is associated with increased risk for comorbidities, such as heart disease, hypertension, chronic respiratory diseases, cancer, and diabetes mellitus, these illnesses were greatly associated with increased risk of severe illness and mortality due to COVID-19 (NICD & NDoH, 2022). During South Africa's third wave of the COVID-19 disease in September 2021, the age groups with the highest cumulative incidence risk were between 50 and 60 years and aged ≥80 years (Naidoo et al., 2022). The estimated natural causes among older people between 3 May 2020 and 30 October 2021 was 198,600 when compared to 69,500 deaths from natural deaths among those younger than 60 years (Naidoo et al., 2022).

There was also an increase in the psycho-social strain on older persons caused by the COVID-19 pandemic. This was particularly due to changes in their daily routine, such as increased isolation and time spent at home, reduced social and physical interaction with family members and friends, temporary or permanent end of employment, as well as anxiety due to the fear of illness and death (WHO, 2020). Social distancing, self-isolation, and staying at home where possible were the primary prevention methods used to curb the infection and spread of COVID-19 (Morley & Vellas, 2020). Nonetheless, loneliness caused by social distancing and isolation among older persons was a major challenge and was linked to increased depression, cognitive dysfunction, disability, cardiovascular disease, and increased mortality (Morley & Vellas, 2020).

Access to Healthcare

As people transition to older ages there is a greater demand for healthcare services. Increased longevity is associated with a higher prevalence of chronic diseases. The well-being of older people is also heavily dependent on their active or passive use of health services (Golomski, 2017). Almost half of the older population rely on public facilities for their healthcare needs (Statistics South Africa, 2018, 2022b). The percentage of older persons who used public facilities increased slightly between 2017 and 2021, while the use of other health facilities dropped (Statistics South

Africa, 2023a). The combination of several issues such as resource scarcity in the public health system and in people's livelihoods, poor transportation networks organised around healthcare, and families split up between rural homes and urban areas have all led people to make unconventional healthcare access decisions (Neely & Ponshunmugam, 2019). Older people are most likely to walk or use public transportation to get to a health facility. Some of the barriers in accessing healthcare for older people include fiscal and transport poverty, crime, and poor infrastructure (van Biljon & van Niekerk, 2021). As people age and become frail, they experience physical difficulties with accessing transport and the long waiting time at healthcare facilities.

There is a high level of disparity among older people in terms of access to medical aid. Nationwide, in total, there are 83 schemes, of which 23 are open and 60 restricted (Golomski, 2017). By the end of 2015, there were collectively almost 4 million main members and 9 million beneficiaries (main members plus dependents), with a pensioner ratio, or percentage of total scheme members over the age of 65, of 7.1%, or approximately 640,000 older individuals (Council for Medical Schemes, 2016). Schemes pay providers on a fee-for-service basis, but members still pay high out-of-pocket costs (Golomski, 2017). Access to medical aid or private health insurance by older persons dropped by 0.5% points between 2017 and 2021 from approximately 23.8% in 2017 to 23.3% in 2021 (Statistics South Africa, 2023a).

The percentage of older persons who were covered by a medical aid or medical benefit scheme or other types of private health insurance was highest among Whites (73.5% in 2017 and 75.7% in 2021) and Indians (31.6% in 2017 and 47.1% in 2021) (Statistics South Africa, 2023a). This largely reflects the disproportional representation of older Whites in having access to medical care. The other groups (Black Africans and Coloureds) were less likely to be covered by a medical aid, medical benefit scheme, or other private health insurance. Between 2017 and 2021, Black African and Coloured older persons experienced a drop in medical aid coverage, while the opposite was observed for other population groups. In 2017, approximately 6.2% of older Black Africans and 18.1% older Coloureds were members of medical aid schemes or private health insurance. This dropped by 0.8% and 2.4% by 2021, respectively

(Statistics South Africa, 2018, 2022b, 2023a). In terms of gender disparities among the total older population, medical age coverage was slightly higher among older women than older men in both years. While older men had higher coverage than older women between 2017 and 2021, they recorded a decrease in medical aid coverage while the coverage for older women remained the same.

Crime

The sense of safety and security among older people is a widely acknowledged factor for policy and practice in age-friendly environments (Van Hoof et al., 2022). Older people may be particularly vulnerable to crimes such as burglary, mugging, petty thievery, and con artists. Older people fear crime, especially violent crime, and this may cause many to remain isolated in their homes. According to Statistics South Africa's Social Profile of Older Persons, 2017–2021, older South Africans generally feel safer walking alone in their areas during the day rather than at night (Statistics South Africa, 2023a). The Social Profile of Older Persons report highlights that between 2020–2021 and 2021–2022, both older men and women felt less safe at night.

There is also growing concern over the issue of elder abuse as the number of older people increases. Elder abuse is a global public health, human rights, and criminal justice problem that goes beyond socio-economic status and geographic region. Elder abuse is quite common and widespread across South Africa. The most vulnerable older people are usually those living in rural areas, of a lower socio-economic class and tend to be more frail (Kotzé, 2018). Older people in South Africa are also likely to be exposed to the risk of financial abuse especially in relation to the old age pensions, which are the main source of economic security for older people in the country (Lloyd-Sherlock et al., 2014). The majority of older people are cared for in communities and those who are very frail receive care from untrained individuals, increasing their risk of being abused (Kotzé, 2018). This is exacerbated by the absence of skilled social welfare and healthcare personnel to oversee geriatric care and community welfare organisations (Kotzé, 2018).

Conclusion

Over the next few decades, South Africa will experience continuous growth of its ageing population. The ageing population of South Africa is growing at a much faster pace than the majority of countries on the African continent. By the year 2050, the population aged 60 years and over will comprise 16% of the total South African population. Thus, population ageing in the country requires much more focus, as the older population will constitute a substantial and growing share of the total population in the near future.

The profile of the ageing population in South Africa shows that life expectancy is expected to increase steadily. In addition, there will be more older women in South Africa than men, meaning that older women will have a higher life expectancy than men. In terms of geographical location, older people are unevenly dispersed between provinces. This necessitates more focus in terms of planning and budget, with emphasis on provinces such as Gauteng and the Western Cape where there are the largest increases in the number of older people.

Gender differentials indicate that older men are more likely than older women to be married which have implications for their health as literature points to married older people having better health than those who are unmarried. Furthermore, employment data indicates that men dominate the older workforce, with more men participating in the labour force at older ages than older women. Thus, elderly men are more likely to have a better socio-economic status than women. The increasing feminisation of the older population, along with the prevailing gender inequalities, are likely to act as a barrier to the growth and success of the country, necessitating structured efforts to address this issue.

Older people who live with family or in multi-generational households have a further health and socio-economic advantage over those who live alone as they receive greater support from the economically active population. In terms of educational attainment, older Black Africans have the lowest levels of literacy and education in comparison to other groups. However, these trends are improving over time, with older Black Africans reporting higher levels of education over time.

The increase in the older population calls for an improvement in the health system of South Africa, as more pressure will be put on an already overwhelmed public health sector. It is vital that national governments take the necessary steps to address deficiencies in the health system in order to promote a supportive and sustainable future for older South Africans. Despite efforts to address some of the challenges brought on by an ageing population, the country nevertheless faces a number of socio-economic challenges, which include high unemployment, poverty, social inequality, and limited access to public services. These difficulties continue to overwhelm South Africans, especially the older population group, and will have an impact on quality of life and the economy collectively.

References

Aboyade, O. M., Beauclair, R., Mbamalu, O. N., Puoane, T. R., & Hughes, G. D. (2016). Health-seeking behaviours of older black women living with non-communicable diseases in an urban township in South Africa. *BMC Complementary and Alternative Medicine, 16*(410), 410.

Akokuwebe, M. E., Osuafor, G. N., & Idemudia, E. S. (2024). Prevalence and association of HIV and tuberculosis status in older adults in South Africa: An urgent need to escalate the scientific and political attention to aging and health. *Frontiers in Public Health, 12*, 1245553.

Alexio, M., Dianne, S., & Hellen, V. (2019). Experiences of different household structures' caring for people living with HIV and AIDS in the antiretroviral era: Case study of Nyamakate rural area in Zimbabwe. *Cogent Social Sciences, 5*(1), 1565075.

Borji, H.S. (2013). *Global economic issues of an aging population.* https://www.investopedia.com/articles/investing/011216/4-global-economic-issues-aging-population.asp

Brear, M. R., Manderson, L., Nkovana, T., & Harling, G. (2024). Conceptualisations of "good care" within informal caregiving networks for older people in rural South Africa. *Social Science & Medicine, 344, 116597.*

Calderón-Larrañaga, A., Dekhtyar, S., Vetrano, D. L., Bellander, T., & Fratiglioni, L. (2020). COVID-19: Risk accumulation among biologically and socially vulnerable older populations. *Ageing Research Reviews, 63, 101149.*

Caldwell, J. C., & Caldwell, P. (1993). The South African fertility decline. *Population and Development Review, 19*(2), 225–262.

Carr, D., & Springer, K. W. (2010). Advances in families and health research in the 21st century. *Journal of Marriage and Family, 72*(3), 743–761.

Council for Medical Schemes. (2016). *Annual report 2014/15*. Council for Medical Schemes.

Czaja, S. J. (2016). Long-term care services and support systems for older adults: The role of technology. *American Psychologist, 71*(4), 294–301.

Dalu, M. T., Manyani, A., & Masunungure, C. (2020). Gender inclusivity and development in South African public urban spaces. In R. Massey & A. Gunter (Eds.), *Urban geography in South Africa: Perspectives and theory*. Cham.

De Jong Gierveld, J., De Valk, H., & Blommesteijn, M. (2000). *Living arrangements of older persons and family support in more developed countries*. United Nations Department of Economic and Social Affairs.

Department of Health (DoH). (1998). *South Africa demographic and health survey 1998*. Department of Health.

Edmonds, E. V., Mammen, K., & Miller, D. L. (2005). Rearranging the family? Income support and elderly living. Arrangements in a low-income country. *Journal of Human Resources, 40*(1), 186–207.

Ferreira, M. (2010). *Housing and older people in South Africa*. International Longevity Centre (ILC) South Africa.

Freedman, V. A., Cornman, J. C., Carr, D., & Lucas, R. E. (2019). Time use and experienced wellbeing of older caregivers: A sequence analysis. *The Gerontologist, 59*(5), 441–450.

Geboers, B., Reijneveld, S. A., Koot, J. A., & De Winter, A. F. (2018). Moving towards a comprehensive approach for health literacy interventions: The development of a health literacy intervention model. *International Journal of Environmental Research and Public Health, 15*(6), 1268.

Golomski, C. (2017). Elder care and private health insurance in South Africa: The pathos of race class. *Medical Anthropology, 37*(4), 311–326.

Grey, E., Baber, F., Corbett, E., Ellis, D., Gillison, F., & Barnett, J. (2024). The use of technology to address loneliness and social isolation among older adults: The role of social care providers. *BMC Public Health, 24*(1), 108.

He, W., Aboderin, I., & Adjaye-Gbewonyo, D. (2020). *Africa aging: 2020*. US Government Printing Office.

Hosegood, V. (2009). The demographic impact of HIV and AIDS across the family and household life-cycle: Implications for efforts to strengthen families in sub-Saharan Africa. *AIDS Care, 21*(1), 13–21.

Hsu, T.-L., & Barrett, A. E. (2020). The association between marital status and psychological well-being: Variation across negative and positive dimensions. *Journal of Family Issues, 41*(11), 2179–2202.

Inouye, S. K., Studenski, S., Tinetti, M. E., & Kuchel, G. A. (2007). Geriatric syndromes: Clinical, research and policy implications of a core geriatric concept. *Journal of the American Geriatrics Society, 55*(5), 780–791.

Jennings, E. A., Chinogurei, C., & Adams, L. (2022). Marital experiences and depressive symptoms among older adults in rural South Africa. *SSM-Mental Health, 2*, 100083.

Kotzé, C. (2018). Elder abuse—The current state of research in South Africa. *Frontiers in Public Health, 6*, 358.

Lam, D., Leibbrandt, M., & Ranchhod, V. (2006). *Labour force withdrawal of the elderly in South Africa*. Centre for Social Science Research University of Cape Town.

Lawrence, E. M., Rogers, R. G., Zajacova, A., & Wadsworth, T. (2019). Marital happiness, marital status, health, and longevity. *Journal of Happiness Studies, 20*(5), 1539–1561.

Lloyd-Sherlock, P., Beard, J., Minicuci, N., Ebrahim, S., & Chatterji, S. (2014). Hypertension among older adults in low-and middle-income countries: Prevalence, awareness and control. *International Journal of Epidemiology, 43*(1), 116–128.

Lloyd-Sherlock, P., Penhale, B., & Ayiga, N. (2018). Financial abuse of older people in low and middle-income countries: The case of South Africa. *Journal of Elder Abuse & Neglect, 30*(3), 236–246.

Lombard, A., & Kruger, E. (2009). Older persons: The case of South Africa. *Ageing International, 34*, 119–135.

Maharaj, P., & Roberts, B. (2021). Growing older with dignity: The nature and determinants of quality of life among older people in South Africa. In F. Rojo-Pérez & G. Fernández-Mayoralas (Eds.), *Handbook of active ageing and quality of life: From concepts to applications*. Springer.

Makiwane, M., & Kwizera, S. A. (2006). An investigation of quality of life of the elderly in South Africa, with specific reference to Mpumalanga Province. *Applied Research in Quality of Life, 1*(3), 297–313.

Morley, J. E., & Vellas, B. (2020). COVID-19 and older adult. *The Journal of Nutrition, Health & Aging, 24*(4), 364–365.

Mtshali, M. N. G. (2016). Role reversal of rural black grandparents in South Africa. *Journal of Comparative Family Studies, 47*(3), 369–377.

Naidoo, I., Groenewald, C., Essack, Z., Isaacs, D., Roberts, B., Zuma, K., Reddy, T., Abdelatif, N., Maharaj, P., Dunn, S., & Msomi, N. (2022). *Understanding the demographic, health, psycho-social and economic implications of COVID-19 on older persons in South Africa*. Human Sciences Research Council.

National Academies of Sciences, Engineering, and Medicine. (2022). *Understanding the aging workforce: Defining a research agenda*. The National Academies Press.

National Department of Health (NDoH). (2018). *The first national TB prevalence survey: South Africa 2018*. National Department of Health.

National Institute for Communicable Diseases (NICD) and National Department of Health (NDoH). (2022). *Coronavirus disease 2019 (COVID-19) caused by a novel coronavirus (SARS-CoV-2)*. NICD and NDoH.

Neely, A. H., & Ponshunmugam, A. (2019). A qualitative approach to examining health care access in rural South Africa. *Social Science & Medicine, 230*(6), 214–221.

Nzima, D., & Maharaj, P. (2020). Long-term care for the elderly in sub-Saharan Africa: An analysis of existing models. In P. Maharaj (Ed.), *Health and care in old age in Africa*. Routledge.

OECD. (2020). *Promoting an age-inclusive workforce. Living, learning and earning longer*. OECD Publishing.

Outlioua, S., & Fazouane, A. (2023). Which factors affect the sustainability of pension schemes? *Economic Affairs, 43*(1), 89–108.

Palamuleni, M., Kalule-Sabiti, I., & Makiwane, M. (2007). Fertility and childbearing in South Africa. In A. Y. Amoateng & T. B. Heaton (Eds.), *Families and households in post-apartheid South Africa: Socio-demographic perspectives*. HSRC Press.

Patel, L., & Triegaardt, J. (2008). South Africa: Social security, poverty alleviation and development. In J. Midgley, K. L. Tang, J. Midgley, & K. L. Tang (Eds.), *Social security, the economy and development*. Palgrave Macmillan.

Peltzer, K., Phaswana-Mafuya, N., & Pengpid, S. (2019). Rural–urban health disparities among older adults in South Africa. *African Journal of Primary Health Care and Family Medicine, 11*(1), 1–6.

Pillay, D., & Maharaj, P. (2013). Population ageing in Africa. In P. Maharaj (Ed.), *Aging and health in Africa*. Springer.

Rademeyer, S., & Maharaj, P. (2020). Ageing in Africa: Patterns and trends. In P. Maharaj (Ed.), *Health and care in old age in Africa*. Routledge.

Ralston, M., Jennings, E., & Schatz, E. (2022). Who is at risk? Social support, relationship dissolution, and illness in a rural context. *Sociological Inquiry, 92*(3), 1053–1082.

Ramocha, L. M., Louw, Q. A., & Tshabalala, M. D. (2017). Quality of life and physical activity among older adults living in institutions compared to the community. *South African Journal of Physiotherapy, 73*(1), 1–6.

Roux, A., & Viljoen, D. (2018). Using futures studies methodologies to explore the economic participation of the older cohorts of South Africa's population towards 2030. *Journal of Futures Studies, 23*(1), 5–22.

Schatz, E., Ralston, M., Madhavan, S., Collinson, M. A., & Gómez-Olivé, F. X. (2018). Living arrangements, disability and gender of older adults among rural South Africa. *The Journals of Gerontology: Series B, 73*(6), 1112–1122.

Schulz, R. (2006). *The encyclopaedia of aging*. Springer.

Solanki, G., Kelly, G., Cornell, J., Daviaud, E., & Geffen, L. (2019). Population ageing in South Africa: Trends, impact, and challenges for the health sector. In *South African health review, 2019*. Health Systems Trust.

Solem, P. E., Hauge, L., Hellevik, T., & Herlofson, K. (2023). Older workers and work exit preferences in a digitalized working life. *Nordic Journal of Working Life Studies, 14*(S12), 1–16.

Statistics South Africa. (2018). *General household survey 2017: Statistical release*. Statistics South Africa.

Statistics South Africa. (2019). *Mid-year population estimates, 2019*. Statistics South Africa.

Statistics South Africa. (2022a). *Census 2022: Statistical release*. Statistics South Africa.

Statistics South Africa. (2022b). *General household survey 2021: Statistical release*. Statistics South Africa.

Statistics South Africa. (2022c). *Mid-year population estimates, 2022*. Statistics South Africa.

Statistics South Africa. (2023a). *The social profile of older persons, 2017–2021*. Statistics South Africa.

Statistics South Africa. (2023b). *Quarterly Labour Force Survey (QLFS), quarter 4: 2023*. Statistics South Africa.

Statistics South Africa. (2024). *Quarterly Labour Force Survey (QLFS), quarter 3: 2024*. Statistics South Africa.

Swartz, L. (2009). *Fertility transition in South Africa and its implications on the four major population groups* (United Nations population bulletin, nos. 48–49). United Nations.

Tesfa, D., Tiruneh, S. A., Gebremariam, A. D., Azanaw, M. M., Engidaw, M. T., Kefale, B., Abebe, B., Dessalegn, T., & Tiruneh, M. (2023). The pooled estimate of the total fertility rate in sub-Saharan Africa using recent (2010–2018) Demographic and Health Survey data. *Frontiers in Public Health, 10*, 1053302.

Thornton, A. (2023). *Household formation, living alone, and not getting married in South Africa* (Working paper number 295). Southern Africa Labour and Development Research Unit.

Tshaka, A., Tanga, P., & Ntshongwana, Z. (2023). Socio-economic challenges experienced by widows and support provided by social workers in Raymond Mhlaba Local Municipality in Eastern Cape, South Africa. *Southern African Journal of Social Work and Social Development, 35*(3), 21.

Tondini, A., Ardington, C., & Woolard, I. (2017). *Public pensions and elderly informal employment: Evidence from a change in retirement age in South Africa* (Working paper number 206). Southern Africa Labour and Development Research Unit.

United Nations Educational, Scientific and Cultural Organization (UNESCO). (2021). *SDG indicator metadata*. UNESCO.

United Nations. (2022). *World population prospects 2022*. United Nations, Department of Economic and Social Affairs, Population Division.

van Biljon, H. M., & van Niekerk, L. (2021). Community mobility and transport use of urban older adults who attend public healthcare in Gauteng, South Africa. *South African Journal of Occupational Therapy, 51*(3), 34–41.

van de Water, B., Abuelezam, N., Hotchkiss, J., Botha, M., & Ramangoaela, L. (2023). The effect of HIV and antiretroviral therapy on drug-resistant tuberculosis treatment outcomes in Eastern Cape, South Africa: A Cohort Study. *Viruses, 15*(11), 2242.

Van Hoof, J., Dikken, J., van Staalduinen, W. H., van der Pas, S., van den Hoven, R. F., & Hulsebosch-Janssen, L. M. (2022). Towards a better understanding of the sense of safety and security of community-dwelling older adults: The case of the age-friendly city of The Hague. *International Journal of Environmental Research and Public Health, 19*(7), 3960.

Velkoff, V. A. (2001). *Living arrangements and well-being of the older population: Future research directions*. United Nations, Department of Economic and Social Affairs, Population Division.

Waite, L. J. (2004). *Aging, health, and public policy: Demographic and economic perspectives*. Population Council.

World Health Organization (WHO). (2015). *World report on ageing and health*. WHO.

World Health Organization (WHO). (2020). *WHO methods and data sources for life tables 1990–2019*. WHO.

World Health Organization (WHO). (2022). *Newsroom ageing and health*. World Health Organization.

Yelin, D., Wirtheim, E., Vetter, P., Kalil, A. C., Bruchfeld, J., Runold, M., Guaraldi, G., Mussini, C., Gudiol, C., Pujol, M., & Bandera, A. (2020). Long-term consequences of COVID-19: Research needs. *The Lancet Infectious Diseases, 20*(10), 1115–1117.

3

Ageing in a Time of Adversity: Personal Wellbeing of Older People in South Africa

Benjamin Roberts and Pranitha Maharaj

Abstract This chapter examines the determinants of personal wellbeing among South Africans aged 60 years and older, using representative data from the South African Social Attitudes Survey (SASAS) covering 2009–2023. Wellbeing increased from 2009 to 2013 but declined steadily from 2016 to 2021, with a slight recovery in 2021–2023. Religion, personal relationships, and community belonging were highly rated domains. However, concerns about health, safety, and financial security remained,

B. Roberts (✉)
Developmental, Capable and Ethical State (DCES) Research Division, Human Sciences Research Council, Durban, South Africa

Institute of Social and Economic Research (ISER), Rhodes University, Makhanda, South Africa
e-mail: BRoberts@hsrc.ac.za

P. Maharaj
School of Built Environment and Development Studies, University of KwaZulu-Natal, Durban, South Africa
e-mail: Maharajp7@ukzn.ac.za

P. Maharaj (ed.), *Navigating Ageing in South Africa*, Sustainable Development Goals Series, https://doi.org/10.1007/978-981-97-9088-3_3

especially among the most vulnerable. Significant disparities in wellbeing exist among older persons, linked to education, employment, and subjective poverty. Higher education levels and employment status correlated with increased life satisfaction, while self-rated poverty significantly reduced wellbeing. Marital status also influenced satisfaction levels. Racial and geographic disparities were evident, with Black African and rural-based older adults displaying lower wellbeing. The analysis also highlights the growing impact of digital technology, with Internet usage enhancing wellbeing, though a digital divide persists. In the context of widespread poverty and socio-economic challenges, the analysis underscores the need for comprehensive social policies focused on elder care, social assistance, healthcare, and digital inclusion to reduce inequalities and improve the quality of life of older South Africans.

Keywords Ageing • Personal wellbeing • Adversity • Life satisfaction • South Africa

Introduction

South Africa is a relatively youthful country, but the population aged 60 years and older is growing rapidly (Statistics South Africa, 2023). This requires a comprehensive social policy approach to ensure that citizens can grow older with dignity, security, and a decent quality of life. Increasingly, the emphasis is not only on living longer but on 'ageing well' in later life. In more developed countries, this changing focus has been accompanied by a shift from measuring 'ageing well' as the absence of disease and illness to assessing what is commonly referred to as subjective wellbeing (Jivraj et al., 2014). Subjective wellbeing is an individual's personal assessment of overall life satisfaction. It is a subjective measure that relies on individuals' self-reported accounts of own thoughts and feelings about their wellbeing (Diener & Suh, 1997). Wellbeing is a vital aspect of quality of life, and its measurement and monitoring is particularly relevant for bringing about improvements in the lives of older people (Møller & Ferreira, 1992). An extensive review of studies on wellbeing reveals several variables, themes, and domains that contribute towards explaining overall life satisfaction, including employment, education, health, marital status, safety, and environmental factors (Diener & Suh, 1997; Reich et al., 2020; Voukelatou et al., 2019).

Health is an essential element of wellbeing and is perhaps one of the main contributors to life satisfaction in later life (Møller, 1993). As people live to an older age, they are more likely to experience a deterioration in their health, which may require medication and sometimes specialised treatment, and which can result in correspondingly low reported levels of personal wellbeing. Older people are also more likely to experience a greater burden of morbidity and disease. They are more prone to suffer from a range of chronic, non-communicable infections, including diabetes, hypertension, heart disease, stroke, and respiratory disorders. Some types of disabilities also increase with age, including hearing and visual impairments. As health declines, frailty and disability become more common, resulting in a greater reliance on external sources for support. A rise in health ailments can disrupt normal daily functioning, significantly affecting quality of life.

Most studies that examine the relationship between subjective wellbeing and marital status find that married individuals report significantly higher levels of life satisfaction than those who are single, separated, divorced, or widowed (Botha & Booysen, 2013; Wadsworth, 2016). Marriage often provides greater financial and emotional support. As people age, loneliness becomes more prevalent due to changes in the quality and quantity of their social relationships (Phaswana-Mafuya & Peltzer, 2017). In their study, Ntozini and Abdullahi (2021) found that loneliness negatively impacts the wellbeing of older adults, with higher levels of loneliness associated with lower levels of wellbeing. Older adults may also find it difficult to sustain social relationships, which can result in social withdrawal and a decline in subjective wellbeing. A multivariate analysis of a nationally representative sample (n = 3624) of older South Africans who took part in the Study of Global Ageing and Adults Health (SAGE) wave 1 found that the prevalence of loneliness among older adults in South Africa is high (Peltzer & Phaswana-Mafuya, 2013). Older people with good subjective health were less likely to experience loneliness than those with poor health. Similarly, those with good cognitive functioning were much less likely to experience loneliness than those with poor cognitive functioning (Peltzer & Phaswana-Mafuya, 2013). Withdrawal from social relations and activities can lead to detachment from mainstream society and may subsequently result in social exclusion (Walsh et al., 2017). Multiple studies have shown that individuals with stronger social networks and more frequent interactions tend to experience higher levels of subjective wellbeing and feel happier when in the company of others (Amati et al., 2018; Walsh et al., 2017).

Regarding racial differences, a South African study undertaken by Kopylova et al. (2022) found that the quality of life of older people varies substantially by race group, with Black Africans significantly less satisfied with their lives than the other race groups. However, the quality of life of Black African adults increased over time, probably related to the historical inequalities created by the apartheid system. Family ties are often crucial for the wellbeing of older adults, representing a core source of social support, especially in the absence of institutional support. In South Africa, family members are often the main source of support in older ages. A majority of older adults reside with their children or other relatives, with slightly more than half staying in extended family households (Statistics South Africa, 2023). A study found that older people with close family ties had better mental health and were also more likely to participate in social activities. Social activities included any of the following: visiting family or friends, attending religious services, going to clubs or organised activities, and going out for enjoyment (Patterson & Margolis, 2023). Older people involved in social activities are less likely to feel lonely and isolated. However, traditional family support is increasingly declining due to changes in family structures resulting from migration, urbanisation, HIV and AIDS, as well as other factors. One consequence of this change is that older adults can no longer rely on guaranteed family assistance. Many anticipated that their children would care for them in their later years, but as their children relocate for economic opportunities or other motivations, they face a situation where this crucial support is lacking.

Employment is another crucial component of wellbeing, since it is likely to provide economic and societal benefits that contribute to people's quality of life. Research from other parts of the world suggests that employment for older people has a range of benefits beyond productivity and economic growth. Working beyond retirement age can yield mental and psychological benefits for older people (Baxter et al., 2021). However, health ailments may increase with age, affecting their ability to remain in employment. As people live longer, they are less likely to be in paid employment. Studies in South Africa suggest that older people, especially those older than 50 years, are less likely to be employed (Riumallo-Herl et al., 2019). For many older people, the government-funded non-contributory old age grant is their main source of income. Schatz et al. (2012) found that the old age grant improves financial wellbeing, but the impact on subjective wellbeing is gendered and transitory. According to the study, wellbeing for recently pension-eligible women (aged 60–64 years) was higher than women in the pre-pension-eligible category (age 55–59 years). A study by Kollamparambi and Etinzock (2019) suggests that the state pension has a positive and significant effect on the wellbeing of women recipients, but not men. However, using the National Income Dynamics Study dataset, Kopylova et al. (2022) found that while the extensive social security system makes older people feel more secure, economic status has a greater impact on wellbeing than other dimensions because of the risk of rising costs of living and more limited options for continued income. Evidence also suggests that the real value of the old age grant is not keeping pace with the cost of living, signifying that this source of support alone is insufficient to meet the care needs of older persons (Moore, 2024).

Research suggests that environmental factors may also have an influence on wellbeing. In her study using the WHO Study of Global Ageing and Adult Health (WHO-SAGE) survey data, Ralston (2018) found that older people living in more resource-deprived areas reported lower subjective wellbeing. Controlling for individual and district-level factors, the analysis revealed that community-level provision of basic services (i.e., water, sanitation, electricity, housing) had a modest but not insignificant impact on the subjective wellbeing of older persons. While South Africa has made significant improvement in the provision of water supply and sanitation services since the end of apartheid, many backlogs and challenges remain.

A safe living environment has been identified as critical for individual wellbeing. Being in a safe living environment has repeatedly been shown to be associated with mental and physical health and higher levels of wellbeing (Putrik et al., 2019). Safety was an important dimension that contributed significantly to the quality of life of older adults in a study conducted in South Africa (Kopylova et al., 2022). This is not surprising, given the high levels of crime in society. High frequencies of homicide, robberies, or substance abuse in the neighbourhood had a significant impact on the wellbeing of individuals. The study found that the heightened risk of being a victim of a crime caused older people to feel more vulnerable, which impacted their wellbeing (Kopylova et al., 2022).

This chapter builds on the research on personal wellbeing undertaken by Maharaj and Roberts (2021). However, it extends the analysis to explore the pattern of, and trends in, the personal wellbeing of South Africans aged 60 years and older. Use is made of fourteen representative social survey rounds covering the period between 2009 and 2023, including data from five additional annual survey rounds beyond that examined by Maharaj and Roberts (2021) in their analysis of the survey for 2009 through 2017, and importantly covering the COVID-19 years and its aftermath. The analysis begins with a presentation of the general level of satisfaction with personal wellbeing and select sub-domains on average over the period, as well as year-on-year changes in evaluation. This is followed by an examination of socio-economic as well as demographic predictors of the personal wellbeing of older people. Finally, the analysis draws on data from the 2017, 2021, and 2022 International Social Survey Programme (ISSP) modules fielded in the South African Social Attitudes Survey (SASAS) on the themes of social networks, health, and the digital society to provide special insight into additional factors that may have a bearing on the wellbeing of older persons in South Africa. The chapter concludes with a review of the survey evidence and its implications for efforts directed at ensuring that all South Africans have an opportunity of 'ageing well', despite adverse contextual conditions.

Methodology

Survey Description

For this study, repeat cross-sectional data from SASAS was used. This nationally representative survey series has been conducted annually by the Human Sciences Research Council (HSRC) since 2003. For the analysis of the pattern and predictors of the personal wellbeing of older persons in South Africa, data from 14 annual rounds of the survey undertaken between 2009 and 2023 were pooled. Each SASAS round involved drawing a random probability sample representative of South Africans aged 16 years and older residing in private households. Respondents were selected through strict random probability methods at every stage of sampling. The Population Census served as the sampling frame, from which 500 small area layers (SALs) were drawn as primary sampling units, with probability proportional to size. In the second stage of sampling, seven dwelling units (or visiting points) were selected with equal probability within each drawn SAL. In the final stage, an individual was selected with equal probability from all eligible persons within the chosen dwelling units. Eligibility was based on age (16 years and older) and residence (having resided at the visiting point at least 14 days in the month prior to interview).

In each SASAS round, a sample of 3500 potential respondents meeting the eligibility criteria was selected, with a target minimum effective sample size of 2500. The realised sample for each annual round over the 2009–2023 period ranged between 2521 and 3305. Data were weighted to account for the relative selection probabilities at the three main sampling stages and benchmarked against the most-recent mid-year population estimates released by Statistics South Africa. The analysis that follows focuses on personal wellbeing patterns among SASAS respondents aged 60 years and older across the 14 survey rounds, resulting in a combined sample of 8178 adults. This combined sample includes annual subsamples of older persons ranging between 413 and 707 respondents in each survey round. The characteristics of the pooled sample of older persons are shown Table 3.1.

Table 3.1 Sample characteristics of older adults aged 60 years and older, 2009–2023

	Pooled sample of older adults aged 60 years and older, 2009–2023, unweighted N and weighted %	
	Unweighted N	Weighted %
All older persons 60 years and older	8178	100.0
Age group		
60–67 years	4230	50.8
68–75 years	2587	30.9
Older than 75 years	1361	18.3
Gender		
Male	3173	45.7
Female	5003	54.3
Population group		
Black African	3694	65.0
Coloured	1388	10.3
Indian/Asian	1346	5.0
White	1744	19.8
Marital status		
Married	3664	51.0
Widowed	2924	32.7
Separated/divorced	542	6.1
Never married	836	10.3
Household size		
1	1693	10.0
2	2605	25.0
3	1329	16.4
4+	2551	48.7
Educational attainment		
Primary or no formal schooling	3161	46.0
Incomplete secondary schooling	2465	28.0
Matric or equivalent	1368	15.0
Tertiary	926	11.0
Employment status		
Employed	675	8.9
Unemployed	579	9.1
Pensioner	6226	77.6

(continued)

Table 3.1 (continued)

	Pooled sample of older adults aged 60 years and older, 2009–2023, unweighted N and weighted %	
	Unweighted N	Weighted %
Other labour inactive	451	4.4
Subjective poverty status		
Poor	1655	23.9
Just getting by	3053	39.5
Non-poor	3399	36.6
Type of geographic location		
Urban areas	6224	68.2
Rural areas	1954	31.8

Source: HSRC SASAS 2009–2023

Face-to-face surveying was undertaken in the last quarter of each year using paper-and-pencil interviewing (PAPI) until 2017 and computer-assisted personal interviewing (CAPI) thereafter, with fieldwork lasting approximately 6 weeks. Participation in the study was entirely voluntary. Respondents were given the assurance of anonymity and they were required to indicate their willingness to participate in the survey by signing consent forms. Ethical approval for the study was obtained from the HSRC's Research Ethics Committee.

Measures

For our analysis of wellbeing, we draw primarily on the Personal Wellbeing Index (PWI, Cummins et al., 2003), using eight standard constituent domains including standard of living, achievement in life, health, safety, future security, personal relationships, feeling part of their community, and spirituality or religion. All these domains have been used as a core measure in the SASAS series since the 2009 round, which allowed for pooling of multiple cross-sectional rounds into a combined file to investigate the wellbeing of older adults over nearly a decade-and-a-half. In addition, we use the single-item satisfaction with life scale (SWL) together with the PWI items. In our analysis we use the PWI and its constituent domains, as well as the SWL measure as dependent variables to examine the quality of life of older adults. Our independent variables include select socio-economic and demographic characteristics, namely age, sex, marital status, household size, employment status, educational attainment, type of geographic location, and subjective poverty status.

Results

Pattern of Personal Wellbeing Among Older Persons

The average PWI score for South Africans aged 60 years and older was 61.7 (±16.7) over the 2009–2023 period, with index values varying between a low of 53.8 and a high of 68.2 for this age group over the course of the 14-year interval. The Cronbach α coefficient for the PWI domain items was 0.85 on aggregate across all years, with only modest variation between 0.81 and 0.88 observed based on year-by-year testing. This level of reliability consistently exceeds the accepted minimum threshold of 0.70. The PWI displayed a strong correlation with "satisfaction with life as a whole" ($r = 0.71$, with a year-by-year range of 0.65–0.77). The PWI item homogeneity index, which is the average of the inter-item correlation coefficients, was 0.41 and the corrected item-total correlations (CITC) varied between 0.45 and 0.73, which exceed the suggested minimum threshold of 0.30 (Rodriguez-Blazquez et al., 2011).

To establish the construct validity of the PWI measure, a bivariate correlation as well as a multiple linear regression was undertaken of the eight PWI domains against the single-item satisfaction with life as a whole item. The findings of this analysis (Table 3.2) revealed that all PWI items were significantly correlated with the SWL measure (r value range: 0.31–0.75). Most PWI domains made a significant unique contribution to overall life satisfaction, apart from personal safety and 'spirituality or religion' domains. The combined unique and shared variance of the PWI domains accounted for 61 percent of the total variance in life satisfaction. The largest unique contribution was made by the living standards domain

Table 3.2 Bivariate correlation and regression of the eight PWI domains on satisfaction with life as a whole for older South African adults aged 60 years and older, pooled 2009–2023 data

	Correlation with 'satisfaction with life as a whole'	Regression: 'satisfaction with life as a whole' as dependent variable		
		B coefficients	Beta coefficients	sr^2 (a)
Satisfaction with:				
1. Standard of living	0.75 ***	0.51***	0.49	0.102
2. Health	0.48 ***	0.06**	0.06	0.002
3. Life achievement	0.65 ***	0.17***	0.16	0.010
4. Personal relationships	0.48 ***	0.06**	0.06	0.002
5. Personal safety	0.39 ***	0.02	0.02	0.000
6. Feeling part of the community	0.43 ***	0.10***	0.09	0.005
7. Future (financial) security	0.52 ***	0.05**	0.05	0.002
8. Spirituality or religion	0.31 ***	0.03	0.03	0.001

* $p<0.05$; ** $p<0.01$; *** $p<0.001$; (ns): not significant; R^2: 0.6089; Adjusted R^2: 0.6085; Total explained unique variability: 0.1235; Total explained shared variability: 0.4854

(a) sr^2 (part coefficient squared): amount of unique variance contributed by each PWI domain

Source: HSRC SASAS 2009–2023

(0.102), followed by the life achievement (0.010) and community connectedness (0.005) domains. The eight domains formed a single factor that explained 48.9% of the variance among older persons in South Africa.

Altogether, the analysis suggests that the PWI has acceptable psychometric properties among older adults in a diverse society such as South Africa. It continues to represent a useful multidimensional tool for examining quality of life among this subpopulation.

In Fig. 3.1, the mean scores for the Personal Wellbeing Index, overall life satisfaction, and the eight PWI domains over the 2009–2023 period on aggregate are presented, ranked in descending order. Only three domains were rated by older persons as providing satisfaction levels

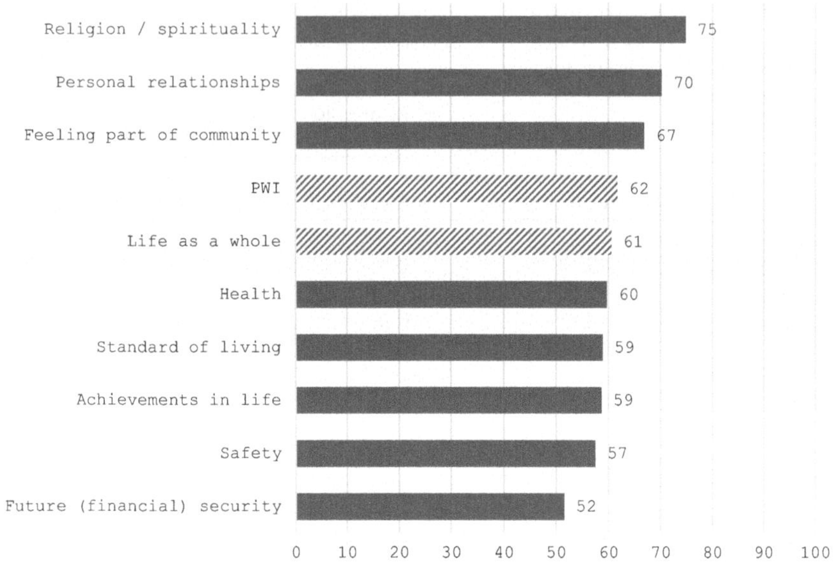

Fig. 3.1 Average PWI and PWI domain scores for older South African adults aged 60 years and older, pooled 2009–2023 data (mean scores based on a 0–100 scales). Source: HSRC SASAS 2009–2023

exceeding the overall PWI and life satisfaction score values (61–62), namely, religion and spirituality (75), personal relationships (70), and feeling part of one's community (67). It is notable that factor analysis based on the pooled data (results not shown) suggests that these three domains cluster together to form a distinct factor separate from the other five domains for older persons in South Africa. They share a common emphasis on social connections, emotional and moral support, a sense of belonging and purpose, and coping and resilience. During the COVID-19 pandemic and beyond, these elements have proven to be crucial factors for the personal wellbeing of older persons.

Apart from these top three ranked domains, more moderate levels of satisfaction were observed for health (60), standard of living (59), and achievements in life (59). The moderate satisfaction ratings on these three domains suggest that many older persons are finding ways to maintain a positive outlook, expressing a sense of health, financial security, and pride in what they have accomplished in life. This may reflect inequalities in circumstance between older persons, which is explored later in the chapter. The final two personal wellbeing domains, safety (57) and future financial security (52), received distinctly lower satisfaction ratings from older persons.

Trends in the Personal Wellbeing of Older Persons, 2009–2023

A limitation of the results described above is that they are based on multi-year averages, which masks the dynamics in personal wellbeing and its dimensions over the past 15 years. They also do not compare the evaluations of quality of life among older persons to those of younger adults. This is important in understanding whether there are appreciable differences between older and younger citizens in South Africa that policy and programmatic interventions may need to take account of. For this reason, the scores for the personal wellbeing domains were run on a year-by-year basis covering the 14-year period and analysed dichotomously for those above and below the 60-year threshold. This was also replicated for the overall PWI measure. The results are presented in a series of line graphs in Fig. 3.2.

Regarding the overall PWI trends over the observed period, there was an initial increase in personal wellbeing among older persons, rising from a low (all-period) base of 54 in 2009 to 63 in 2011. After levelling off in 2012, satisfaction rose further to 68 in 2013. A more fluctuating pattern was evident between 2013 and 2016 at generally high levels, with a short-lived decline in wellbeing between 2013 and 2014 being followed by a gradual return to the 2013 peak over the 2014–2016 period. The wellbeing of older persons then entered a sustained period of decline between 2016 and 2021, with PWI scores dropping from 68 in 2016 to 58 in 2021. A slight recovery was observed in 2021–2023, with satisfaction scores stabilising at around 60. Over the 2018–2023 period, wellbeing was relatively flat, with scores in the 58–60 score range. It is interesting to observe that there was not a decisive decline in the wellbeing of older

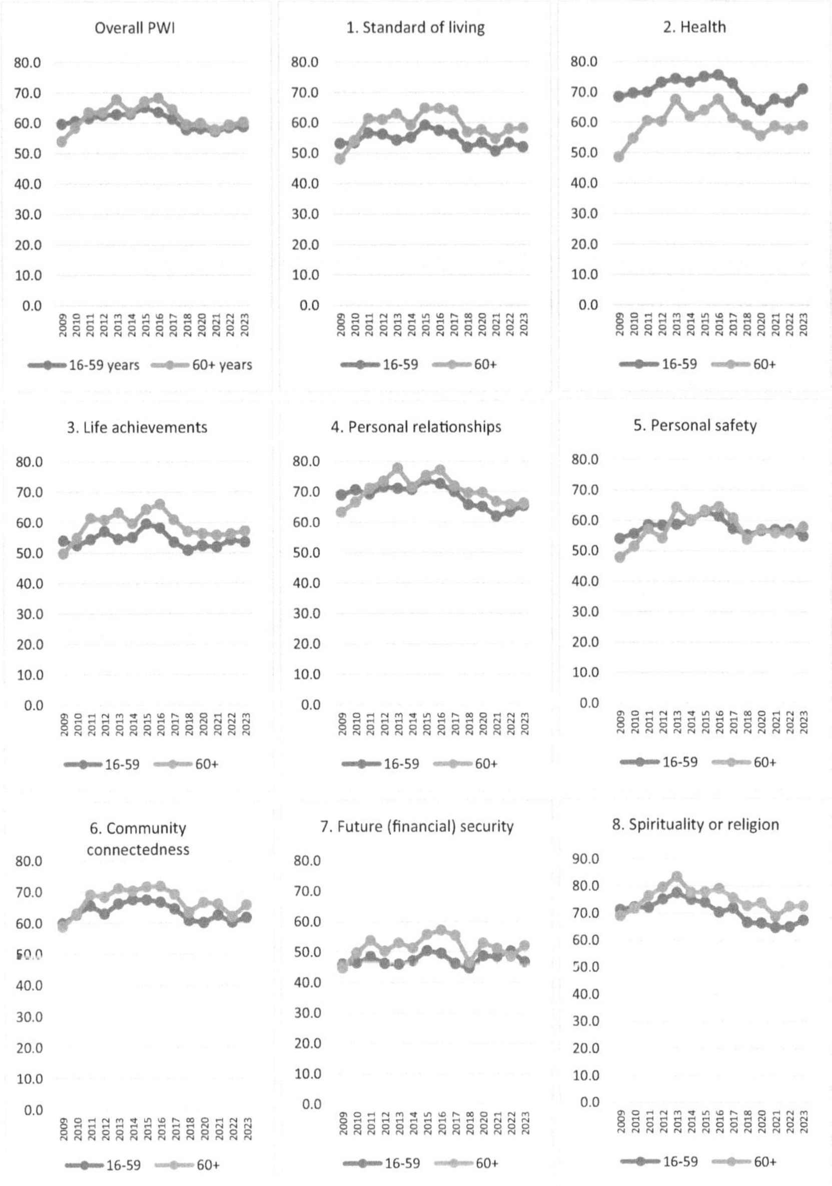

Fig. 3.2 Trends in PWI and PWI domain scores for South Africans aged 60 years and older in comparison to those 16–59 years, 2009–2023 (mean scores based on a 0–100 scales). Source: HSRC SASAS 2009–2023

persons during the COVID-19 pandemic and associated lockdown period of 2020–2021. There was a negligible downturn in 2021 relative to 2020 (-1), but this pales in comparison to the reversal that occurred between 2016 and 2018 (-9).

Comparing the above PWI trends to those of 16–59-year-olds, it is apparent that both younger and older age groups experienced fluctuations in their personal wellbeing between 2009 and 2023. However, older adults consistently reported slightly higher satisfaction levels overall, except for 2009–2010. Both groups showed a trend of initial improvement, followed by a period of decline, and then a modest recovery towards the end of the period. In the case of 16–59-year-olds, the scale of improvement between 2009 and 2015 was more gradual than older persons, with PWI scores rising from 60 to 65. The subsequent period of downturn (2015–2018) occurred 2 years earlier, suggesting that 2015 and 2016 were more difficult years for younger adults relative to older persons. The difference in PWI values between the two age groups in the period of levelling out and slight recovery over 2019–2023 is nominal, with an average PWI score difference of only 1.3 on the 0–100 scale.

Turning to the trends for the specific personal wellbeing domains that make up the PWI, most domains displayed a distinct improvement from 2009 to the mid-2010s for older persons. This was followed by periods of decline, as well as stabilisation or slight recovery in recent years. Of particular concern are the aspects of health, safety, and future security, which tended to show more variability on average and may therefore require targeted policy interventions and community support to ensure that they become more resilient and stable in the face of contextual change. The trend analysis again points to the role of social factors in the lives of older persons. The strong and relatively stable emphasis on personal relationships and community integration suggests that these are key factors contributing to the wellbeing of older persons, highlighting the importance of social support systems. Similarly, religion and spirituality remained a consistently robust source of satisfaction for older persons, reflecting its importance to their overall sense of wellbeing. Personal relationships, community connectedness, and spirituality/religion have, however, not been immune to recent declining patterns and will have contributed to the aggregate PWI decline and levelling off experienced since the late 2020s.

Comparing the trends for older persons with those for individuals aged 16–59 years, the first and most obvious observation is the general similarity in the overall trend pattern between the age groups over the 2009–2023 period across the different personal wellbeing domains. A notable finding is that health satisfaction among those aged 16–59 is consistently higher than for those aged 60 and older. This is the only domain where satisfaction among 16–59-year-olds significantly surpasses that of older persons. On average, the difference in scores between the two groups is 11 points on the 0–100 scale. Health satisfaction is also somewhat more stable for those aged 16–59 years, even though both age groups experienced a decline after the mid-2010s, followed by a modest recovery after 2020. Satisfaction with personal safety displayed the least amount of variation by age group, with an average difference in scores of just 0.1 over the 2009–2023 period. This suggests a common concern regarding safety across both age groups.

For the other six dimensions, satisfaction among older persons exceeded that of those aged 16–59 years, though the scale of this variation differs in extent:

- *Living standard, life achievements, and spirituality/religion*: Older persons reported higher satisfaction, with an average difference of 4.4 to 4.5 points on the 0–100 scale.
- *Future security and community connectedness*: The differences were more moderate, with average differences of 4.1 and 3.4 points, respectively.
- *Personal relationships*: Satisfaction levels for the two age groups were more similar, with an average difference of 1.8 points. Both groups reported fairly high levels of satisfaction in this domain, highlighting the importance of, and broad contentment with, social connections irrespective of age.

Across most of the domains, the satisfaction levels recorded since 2018 are in many instances the lowest recorded for both age groups since the early 2010s. For those aged 16–59 years, the satisfaction ratings for health, personal relationships, and spirituality/religion during this recent period are the lowest recorded over the 14 years of data collection. The only exception to the above is in respect of future security, where the trend for both age groups is not the lowest recorded in recent years and has fluctuated in a narrow range and at a lower level than other domains. For both age groups, this suggests deep-set worries about outlook and the ability to ensure basic needs are met in future, especially given the increasingly challenging economic times South Africans find themselves in. The fact that personal wellbeing in the other domains, for younger and older persons alike, is the lowest it has been in more than a decade suggests increasing duress on a range of fronts. These challenges will require targeted policy interventions to address the specific needs of both younger and older populations and creates a more supportive environment that allows for improvements in their personal wellbeing to be achieved over time.

Socio-Demographic Differences in Subjective Wellbeing Among Older South Africans

Having established the overall and domain-specific trends in personal wellbeing among older persons since the late 2000s, it is important to consider whether there are distinctive attributes among older persons in South Africa that predispose them to higher or lower levels of wellbeing. In Table 3.3, the pooled older persons data for 2009–2023 is analysed, with mean scores of the PWI and satisfaction with life as-a-whole measures presented across a chosen set of socio-economic and demographic characteristics. The latter is included as a robustness check to determine the consistency of findings across the measure. To assess the statistical significance and patterns of wellbeing differences among older adults, one-way ANOVA and post hoc Scheffe tests were conducted.

In terms of age and wellbeing, older persons over 75 years reported lower PWI scores compared to those aged 60–67 and 68–75 years, though the scale of variation was modest in nature. The slight inverted U-shaped predisposition in wellbeing was evident, with the mean score for 68–75-year-olds marginally higher relative to those in the other two

Table 3.3 Mean PWI and SWL scores for older South African adults aged 60 years and older, by select socio-demographic attributes, pooled 2009–2023 data

	PWI-8			SWL		
	Mean score	Sig.	Post hoc Scheffe	Mean score	Sig.	Post hoc Scheffe
All older persons ≥60 years	61.7	…		60.6	…	
Age group		***	60–67, 68–75 > 75+		***	68–75 > 60–67
60–67 years	61.8			59.8		
68–75 years	62.3			62.2		
Older than 75 years	60.4			60.1		
Gender						
Male	63.4	***	Male > female	61.7	***	Male > female
Female	60.3			59.6		
Population group						
Black African	58.3	***	W, I > C > BA	55.8	***	W, I > C > BA
Coloured	64.4			63.8		
Indian/Asian	68.7			71.6		
White	69.7			72.0		
Marital status						
Married	64.6	***	M > W, S/D > NM	63.3	***	M > W, S/D >NM
Widowed	59.7			59.4		
Separated/divorced	59.2			57.9		
Never married	55.5			51.8		
Household size						
1	61.1	***	(1) 2 > 1, 3, 4+	61.7	***	2 > 1, 3 > 4+
2	65.6			66.3		
3	62.1		(2) 3 > 4+	60.7		
4 or more	59.7			57.4		
Educational attainment						
Primary or no formal schooling	57.8	***	T > M > IS > PNF	56.7	***	T > M > IS > PNF
Incomplete secondary schooling	61.9			59.5		
Matric or equivalent	65.6			63.6		
Tertiary	72.4			75.1		

(*continued*)

Table 3.3 (continued)

	PWI-8			SWL		
	Mean score	Sig.	Post hoc Scheffe	Mean score	Sig.	Post hoc Scheffe
Employment status						
Employed	65.4	***	E > P, OLI > U	64.8	***	(1) E, OLI, P > U
Unemployed	56.7			51.4		(2) E > P
Pensioner	61.8			60.8		
Other labour inactive	61.7			63.1		
Subjective poverty status						
Poor	51.7	***	NP > JGB > P	47.4	***	NP > JGB > P
Just getting by	61.3			59.8		
Non-poor	68.8			69.9		
Type of geographic location						
Urban	63.9	***	U > R	63.6	***	U > R
Rural	57.5			54.2		

Source: HSRC SASAS 2009–2023

age groups. This is apparent on the SWL scale as well as the PWI measure. Older men tended to report higher wellbeing than older women on average. This finding is more distinctive when using the PWI than the SWL measure, yet the size of variation should not be overstated (3.1 vs 2.1 on the 0–100 scale). Compared to age and gender differences, a noticeable racial gradient in wellbeing is evident among older South Africans. The wellbeing scores for older White and Indian adults is significantly higher than older Coloured adults, who in turn have higher PWI scores than older Black African adults. The difference is pronounced, with a 12-point variation on the 0–100 scale between older Black African and White adults (58 vs. 70). This disparity remains even when life satisfaction is used instead of the PWI, highlighting persisting racial inequalities in the country.

Married older persons enjoyed higher wellbeing compared to their never-married counterparts, a finding that was evident using both PWI and SWL measures. Married individuals also reported higher PWI scores than those who were widowed, separated, or divorced. This suggests that living together with another person enhances wellbeing compared to living alone or in households with three or more people. This suggests the importance of partnerships for improved wellbeing among older adults. However, the presence of additional household members beyond a spouse or partner tends to reduce PWI and SWL scores. This reduction may be associated with the challenges that other household members can bring, which can offset the benefits of living with a spouse or partner.

Regarding differences by class, educational attainment stands out as a particularly significant factor influencing wellbeing. Older persons with higher levels of education exhibited substantially higher PWI and SWL scores compared to those with less than tertiary level education. Specifically, older individuals with a tertiary level of education had a higher mean PWI score (14 points) than those with primary-level or no formal education (72 vs. 58), and an 18-point gap on the SWL scale (75 vs. 57). These educational disparities likely influenced life opportunities, leading to appreciable inequalities in the material resources necessary for a comfortable retirement. Employment was also found to significantly boost wellbeing among older persons, highlighting the value of employment opportunities and financial security for this age group. Conversely, unemployed older adults showed lower personal wellbeing compared to those still working, retirees, and others who were labour-inactive, such as homemakers or those permanently sick or disabled.

Subjective poverty status was another crucial determinant of personal wellbeing among older persons. The self-rated poor demonstrated significantly lower satisfaction levels (using both the PWI and SWL measures) compared to those who were just getting by or the non-poor. The average score difference between the poor and non-poor was 17 points on the PWI scale and 23 points on the SWL scale. These results highlight the profound impact that material disadvantage has on the quality of retirement in South Africa. Additionally, spatial disparities were evident, with urban dwellers having higher wellbeing scores than rural residents. This indicates a pressing need for improved services and living conditions in rural areas to bridge this gap.

Collectively, our analysis reveals significant inequalities in personal wellbeing among older adults in South Africans, informed by a range of factors such as age, class, race, gender, marital status, and geographic location. Looking at the mean scores across the older person traits that were included in the analysis (Fig. 3.3), we find the highest PWI scores (range: 68–72) among those with a tertiary education, White and Indian adults, the non-poor, and those residing in the Western Cape. These groups of older persons are likely to benefit from better access to resources, social support, and overall higher living standards. Conversely, the lowest mean PWI scores were found among the poor, the never married, the unemployed, those with primary or no formal schooling, and rural residents. These groups are likely to face greater economic challenges, social isolation, and limited access to essential services, which negatively impact their overall wellbeing. These research findings highlight the multifaceted nature of wellbeing and the need for a comprehensive social policy approach to addressing inequalities among older South Africans.

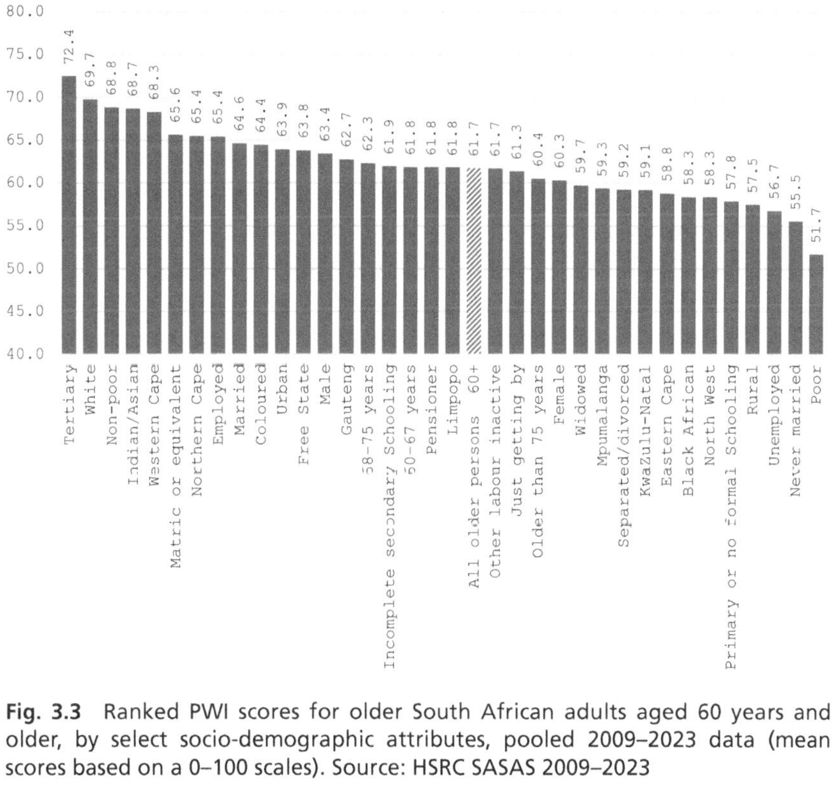

Fig. 3.3 Ranked PWI scores for older South African adults aged 60 years and older, by select socio-demographic attributes, pooled 2009–2023 data (mean scores based on a 0–100 scales). Source: HSRC SASAS 2009–2023

To identify the most influential factors and their combined impact on personal wellbeing, linear regression (OLS) modelling was conducted. The initial model used the PWI-8 measure as the dependent variable and the socio-demographic characteristics mentioned above as independent variables (Table 3.4). An all-year model was run, covering the full 2009–2023 period, after which three separate models were run for three specific aggregated time periods: 2009–2013, 2014–2018, and 2019–2023. Each model controlled for the year of survey, with results that were statistically insignificant (not shown in the table).

In the initial all-year PWI-8 regression model (Model I), gender and age were statistically insignificant predictors. Black African adults had lower PWI scores than White adults, while Coloured adults had slightly higher scores than White adults. Unmarried, separated/divorced, or widowed adults had lower scores than married adults, while having larger numbers of household members moderately reduced wellbeing. There was mixed evidence on a class effect informing the wellbeing of older persons. Those with a secondary or lower level of education had lower PWI scores than those with a tertiary education. There was however no employment status effect evident, implying that working or being in retirement had no bearing on wellbeing, controlling for other variables. Subjective poverty status mattered, with those classifying themselves as poor or vulnerable having lower PWI scores than those who were non-poor. No rural–urban variation was apparent, controlling for other attributes. This model explained around a quarter (24.3%) of variance in the personal wellbeing measure among this older cohort of South Africans.

Models II–IV provide insight into how the relevance and impact of socio-demographic factors on the personal wellbeing among older South African adults evolved over different time periods between 2009 and 2023. The findings suggest that certain factors, such as education level and subjective poverty, remained consistently important, whereas the influence of others, such as race and marital status, varied over time. Being relatively less educated and poorer had a clear negative effect on wellbeing across the three time periods. Being unmarried or separated/divorced displayed a growing negative influence on the wellbeing of older persons over time, especially following COVID-19. The lower wellbeing among Black African adults relative to White adults in 2009–13 and

Table 3.4 Linear regression of socio-demographic attributes on overall PWI scores among older South African adults aged 60 years and older, pooled 2009–2023 data and grouped periods (standardised beta coefficients)

Independent variables (a)	Model I PWI-8 (2009–2023)	Model II PWI-8 (2009–2013)	Model III PWI-8 (2014–2018)	Model IV PWI-8 (2019–2023)
(Constant)	73.42	74.52	78.15	80.72
Female	...	...	...	...
Age (years)	...	...	...	...
Population group (ref.=white)				
Black African	-0.07**	-0.11*	-0.12**	...
Coloured	0.04*	0.09**	...	0.07**
Indian/Asian	...	...	...	...
Marital status (ref=married)				
Widowed	-0.05*	...	...	...
Separated/ divorced	-0.06**	...	-0.06**	-0.08*
Never married	-0.08***	...	-0.07**	-0.11**
Household size	-0.04*	...	...	...
Education level (ref.-tertiary)				
Primary/none	-0.19***	-0.20**	-0.17**	-0.23***
Incompl. secondary	-0.16***	-0.16***	-0.17***	-0.15**
Matric	-0.10***	-0.11***	-0.12***	-0.09*
Employment status (ref=employed)				
Unemployed	...	...	...	...
Pensioner	...	...	...	...
Other inactive	...	...	...	...
Subjective poverty (ref.=non-poor)				
Poor	-0.33***	-0.35***	-0.38***	-0.26***
Just getting by	-0.14***	-0.15**	-0.16***	-0.13***
Geographic location (ref=urban)				
Rural	...	...	...	...

(*continued*)

Table 3.4 (continued)

Independent variables (a)	Model I PWI-8 (2009–2023)	Model II PWI-8 (2009–2013)	Model III PWI-8 (2014–2018)	Model IV PWI-8 (2019–2023)
R^2	0.2425	0.3136	0.2576	0.1521
N	7455	2136	3004	2315

Cells with '...' indicates statistically non-significant variables. Significance is denoted as follows: * p<0.05, **p<0.01, ***p<0.001

(a) Apart from the socio-demographic attributes reported in the table, the models also controlled for year of survey round

Source: HSRC SASAS 2009–2023

2014–18 fell away in 2019–23. Gender, age, employment status, and rural/urban location all remained non-significant predictors of wellbeing among this ageing cohort.

Overall, these results point to the role of class, and to some degree companionship through a life partner, playing a strong role in terms of older person wellbeing. The variation in R^2 values in the models indicates that the explanatory power of socio-demographic variables on life satisfaction fluctuates over time, with Model II having the highest and Model IV the lowest explanatory power. This suggests other factors may increasingly be informing patterns of wellbeing.

Other Factors Associated with the Wellbeing of Older South Africans

As discussed earlier in this chapter, existing literature on quality of life research highlights various factors beyond socio-demographic characteristics that influence personal wellbeing. However, in South Africa, testing the relevance of these factors among older adults is often limited by data availability. Nationally representative surveys that include the PWI generally lack comprehensive measures related to health, social and cultural capital, social participation, and other issues of growing salience, such as digital skills and attitudes towards technology in an increasingly digital society. Recognising this limitation, we draw on in-depth content on these themes included in International Social Survey Programme (ISSP) modules fielded in the 2017, 2021, and 2022 rounds of SASAS.

In this section, we direct attention to key aspects of the themes of social networks, health, and the digital society. These are societal issues that have assumed prominence in recent years, especially due to the multifaceted impacts that the COVID-19 pandemic had on society, and the social changes that continue to occur as a consequence.

Social Networks

Maharaj and Roberts (2021) analysed data from the ISSP module on social networks fielded in SASAS 2017 to determine the relative effects of select constructs on the wellbeing of older persons, using a single-item life satisfaction measure (7-point scale). A summary of salient results is provided here. Feelings of social isolation did not significantly affect life satisfaction, but health variables had a clear impact. Self-efficacy, as measured by a sense that one can accomplish one's goals (i.e., performance accomplishment), had the largest effect, explaining a quarter of variation in the wellbeing of older persons. Depressive mood was inversely correlated with life satisfaction (beta = -0.36), explaining 12.7% of variance, and remained significant even after socio-demographic controls were added (beta = -0.24). Self-efficacy had the largest effect, explaining 24.5% of variance. Better self-reported health also improved wellbeing.

Social capital measures showed mixed results. General contact frequency had no impact on life satisfaction, though face-to-face contact had a weak positive effect that lost significance with socio-demographic controls. Social media use did not affect wellbeing, nor did contact with family or friends. Higher frequency of socialising increased wellbeing, but this effect disappeared once socio-demographic attributes were controlled. Strain and conflict in social relations consistently reduced wellbeing. Cultural capital also influenced wellbeing. Frequent Internet use was positively associated with life satisfaction, suggesting the value of accessing information and staying connected. Public participation in group activities had a positive effect, though this weakened after adding socio-demographic controls. Interpersonal trust showed a modest positive association with wellbeing.

A combined model showed that depressive mood and social strain reduced wellbeing, while self-efficacy, face-to-face contact, and Internet use increased it. Adding socio-demographic attributes left depressive mood, strain, and self-efficacy effects unchanged, but social trust and participation became significant. This model explained close to half the variance in life satisfaction. Overall, the quality of social interactions, health status, and self-efficacy are crucial for the wellbeing of older South Africans.

Health and Healthcare Access

The 2021 SASAS round included the ISSP module on health, allowing us to revisit the 2017 findings in the context of COVID-19, and examine the relationship between health and wellbeing among older persons more comprehensively. Again, a series of OLS regression models were run, containing the influence of single health predictor variables on the dependent life satisfaction variable (0–10 scale), followed by a replication with socio-demographic attributes added. The results in Table 3.5 clustered around the themes of health status, health behaviour, type of healthcare access, and evaluations of local healthcare services.

Regarding health status, a set of five items on functioning, pain, and depression were tested and combined into index form (α = 0.82). Unhappiness and depression, loss of self-confidence, and a lack of self-efficacy were all inversely associated with life satisfaction among older persons in 2021. While this reaffirms the 2017 results, these associations lost significance once socio-demographic attributes were controlled for. This suggests that differences in physical functioning and mental health among older persons are influenced by demographic and class traits. No wellbeing effect was found among older persons based on self-reported health status and long-standing illness, chronic condition, or disability.

A final set of items examined satisfaction with different health care services in one's area of residence. Satisfaction with waiting times, doctor's treatment, and nurse's treatment each showed a significant positive

Table 3.5 Summary of linear regression of health attributes on satisfaction with life among older South African adults aged 60 years and older, 2021 (standardised beta coefficients)

	Model with independent variable only			With additional socio-demographic variables		
Independent variables (1)	Beta coefficient	Sig.	R^2	Beta coefficient	Sig.	R^2
SWL (10-point scale, recoded to 0–100), 2021						
Health status						
Self-reported health status (poor to excellent)	0.00	n.s.	0.0000	-0.08	n.s.	0.1840
Long-standing illness, chronic condition, or disability	0.02	n.s.	0.0006	0.11	n.s.	0.1894
Functioning, pain, and depression index	-0.17	***	0.0297	-0.07	n.s.	0.1832
Difficulties with work or household activities because of health problems	-0.06	n.s.	0.0032	0.03	n.s.	0.1794
Experience of bodily aches or pains	0.00	n.s.	0.0000	0.04	n.s.	0.1803
Feelings of unhappiness and depression	-0.24	***	0.0559	-0.14	n.s.	0.1954
Loss of confidence in themselves	-0.19	***	0.0374	-0.12	n.s.	0.1910
Feeling that they could not overcome problems	-0.19	***	0.0354	-0.10	n.s.	0.1869
Satisfaction with health care services in area						
...the amount of time patients wait before getting served	0.23	***	0.0547	0.10	*	0.1857

(continued)

Table 3.5 (continued)

Independent variables (1)	Model with independent variable only			With additional socio-demographic variables		
	Beta coefficient	Sig.	R^2	Beta coefficient	Sig.	R^2
...the way patients are treated by doctors	0.13	**	0.0178	0.12	**	0.1911
...the way patients are treated by nurses	0.20	***	0.0396	0.11	**	0.1900
...the availability of medicines at the hospital or clinic for both in- and out-patients	0.08	n.s.	0.0064	0.04	n.s.	0.1805
...availability of emergency services such as ambulances and emergency departments at hospitals.	0.16	***	0.0249	0.07	n.s.	0.1824

Source: HSRC SASAS 2021

association with life satisfaction. After controlling for socio-demographic factors, these associations weakened but nonetheless remained significant, indicating that shorter wait times and respectful treatment by healthcare professionals modestly improved life satisfaction, even when accounting for background characteristics. Satisfaction with emergency services had a significant positive association with life satisfaction. However, this relationship became non-significant when socio-demographic factors were controlled for, suggesting that the influence of emergency service satisfaction on life satisfaction is less pronounced once other background characteristics are considered. Finally, satisfaction with the availability of medicines did not have a significant association with life satisfaction.

Digital Society

The 2022 SASAS round included a set of pilot measures related to the ISSP 2024 module on the digital society. Key topics included science and technology (S&T) beliefs, digital access and capabilities, and beliefs about Internet usage, thus revisiting aspects of the 2017 social networks module examined by Maharaj and Roberts (2021). Given that the digital divide is known to reflect generational differences, with older persons generally less likely to have higher digital skills and usage than younger generations, the rapid intensification of digital communication and networking that COVID-19 brought about may have fostered a sense of alienation and loneliness among older persons. Yet, it may also have promoted more regular contact and communication with family and social networks for those able to make the technological leap, thus bolstering wellbeing. The same regression approach was adopted, with the dependent variable being a 5-point life satisfaction item (1–5 scale, recoded to 0–100), with the results outlined in Table 3.6.

In terms of S&T beliefs, there is no statistically significant relationship between the life satisfaction of older persons and a belief that technologies make life easier. However, a negative association ($\beta = -0.15$, $p < 0.01$, $R^2 = 0.0231$) is evident for the belief that technologies are increasing the complexity of life. This association weakens but remains significant when socio-demographic controls are added, suggesting that this belief has a modest pull-down effect on life satisfaction even after considering socio-demographic factors.

As for Internet usage and digital capabilities, a significant positive association was found between the life satisfaction of older persons and frequency of Internet use, and (for those that are Internet users) the ability to use the Internet, use software and apps, and be proficient online. Once socio-demographic controls were added, these associations weakened somewhat and lost significance in the case of frequency of Internet usage. The frequency of Internet usage for specific activities also had a bearing on personal wellbeing. All eight examples tested, ranging from communication with others through to entertainment and financial transactions, produced significant positive effects. The inclusion of socio-demographic

Table 3.6 Summary of linear regression of digital attitudes and behaviour on satisfaction with life among older South African adults aged 60 years and older, 2022 (standardised beta coefficients)

	Model with independent variable only			With additional socio-demographic variables		
Independent variables (1)	Beta coefficient	Sig.	R^2	Beta coefficient	Sig.	R^2
SWL (5-point scale, recoded to 0–100), 2022						
S&T beliefs						
Technologies are making our lives easier and more comfortable	-0.07	n.s.	0.0046	-0.07	n.s.	0.2427
Because of technologies, the world has become far too complex these days	-0.15	**	0.0231	-0.11	*	0.2503
Internet usage and digital skills						
Frequency of Internet usage	0.24	***	0.0533	0.05	n.s.	0.2395
Ability to use the internet (Internet users only)	0.35	***	0.1245	0.20	*	0.3449
Ability to use software or apps (Internet users only)	0.37	***	0.1397	0.22	**	0.3515
Online skills proficiency index (Internet users only)	0.36	***	0.1321	0.23	*	0.3536
Frequency of Internet use for... (all older persons):						
...communicating with others (e.g. messages, social media, email, video chats)	0.26	***	0.0687	0.12	*	0.2397
...sharing or posting photos or videos	0.26	***	0.0702	0.12	*	0.2385

(*continued*)

Table 3.6 (continued)

	Model with independent variable only			With additional socio-demographic variables		
Independent variables (1)	Beta coefficient	Sig.	R^2	Beta coefficient	Sig.	R^2
...creating new content (e.g. web design, blogging, influencing)	0.23	***	0.0535	0.11	*	0.2402
...searching for information	0.32	***	0.1037	0.18	**	0.2491
...gaming	0.15	**	0.0238	0.05	n.s.	0.2324
...downloading or listening to music or watching videos and movies	0.22	***	0.0506	0.10	n.s.	0.2374
...sending money to or receiving money from relatives and friends	0.22	***	0.0493	0.03	n.s.	0.2311
...shopping, paying bills, and other financial transactions	0.26	***	0.0700	0.07	n.s.	0.2330

Source: HSRC SASAS 2022

controls again served to weaken the associations. Communicating with others, sharing/posting photos and videos, creating new online content (e.g., web design, blogging, influencing), and searching for information all retained modest positive associations with life satisfaction of older persons. The effects of online gaming, listening to music or watching videos, sending or receiving money, and shopping or paying bills, however, became statistically non-significant.

A set of beliefs about Internet usage were also tested (data not shown), including the effects of the importance of online connectivity for keeping in touch with others, meeting people online, and avoiding feelings of loneliness. None of these items exerted a significant influence on life satisfaction.

Conclusion

To better understand the pattern and determinants of the personal wellbeing of South Africans aged 60 years and over, this chapter made use of pooled nationally representative South African Social Attitudes Survey (SASAS) data covering a 14-year period. In so doing, it extended the analysis covering 2009–2017 undertaken by Maharaj and Roberts (2021). A number of salient issues emerged from the analysis, which will no doubt require further exploration in future research. Nonetheless, a number of general issues emerged prominently in the study.

Using the Personal Wellbeing Index (PWI) measure, the analysis found that three domains of wellbeing tended to be more highly rated on average by older persons: religion and spirituality, personal relationships, and feeling part of one's community. Religion and spirituality play a salient role in the personal wellbeing of older adults. From a social insurance perspective, religion and spirituality are likely to offer emotional support, moral guidance, coping mechanisms for life's challenges, and a sense of community, all of which are particularly important in later life. The above-average score for personal relationships points to the importance of social connections in the lives of older persons. Strong relationships with family, friends, and significant others provide emotional support and lessen feelings of loneliness, which can serve as a source of joy and security, thereby contributing significantly to their wellbeing. A sense of community belonging appears to be another source of contentment for older persons. Community involvement can provide opportunities for social interaction, support networks, and active participation in communal activities, all of which are beneficial for mental and emotional health.

Apart from these three highly rated domains, other elements including health, standard of living, and achievements in life have an influence on wellbeing. This is probably related to some of the challenges that older persons experience with diminishing physical health, limited financial and material resources, and, by extension, a sense of fulfilment and accomplishment in life. Yet, the moderate satisfaction ratings on these domains also suggest that many older persons are finding ways to maintain a positive outlook, expressing a sense of health, financial security, and pride in what they have accomplished in life. The low scores on the two remaining personal wellbeing domains, safety and future financial security, are likely to reflect concerns about crime and violence, inflation and the rising cost of living, and the ability to meet basic living expenses and unexpected financial needs in future. Health and mobility issues make many older persons more vulnerable to criminal victimisation. In addition, the economic reliance of many on government-provided old age grants as well as family members renders them vulnerable to economic instability and a challenging macroeconomic environment. It is essential that economic and social policy continues to focus on identifying and implementing measures directed at improving the living standards, health services, and personal security of older persons in order to enhance their wellbeing.

With respect to wellbeing trends, there was a distinct increase in PWI scores among older persons between 2009 and 2013, followed by a more fluctuating pattern between 2013 and 2016 at generally high levels. The wellbeing of older persons then entered a sustained period of decline between 2016 and 2021, followed by a slight recovery over the 2021–2023 period. The PWI scores over the 2018–2023 period remained relatively flat and represented the lowest figures in a decade. Similarly, across most of the wellbeing domains, the satisfaction levels recorded over the 2018–2023 period are in many instances the lowest recorded for both age groups since the early 2010s. It is notable that a decisive decline in the wellbeing of older persons was not observed during the COVID-19 pandemic and the lockdown period of 2020–2021, with only a negligible downturn evident relative to the more substantive reversal preceding it from 2016 to 2018.

Older persons generally reported slightly higher satisfaction levels than younger adults, with the exception of 2009–2010. However, health satisfaction among those aged 60 years and older was consistently lower than for those younger than 60. As people age, they are more likely to experience health conditions, which adversely impact their life satisfaction. For both age groups, satisfaction with personal safety was a common concern, which is probably a reflection of the high levels of crime in the country. The oldest age group (75+ years) reported the lowest wellbeing, but there was also a slightly lower mean score among those aged

60–67 years relative to those aged 68–75 years. The lower wellbeing scores for those aged 60–67 may relate to the experience of economic vulnerability in the years immediately after reaching the country's pensionable age (60 years). This is the age that South Africans become eligible to receive the government-provided old-age grant, which is the primary income source for those 60 years and older. Certain initial barriers to accessing grants by some older persons may have led to delayed access and hardship during their early sixties. There is also a significant gender disparity in personal wellbeing among older persons in the country. Older women tended to report lower wellbeing than men on average. Studies have shown that women generally live longer than men, but they may experience relatively more ill health, and this is likely to impact their personal wellbeing (Baum et al., 2021). In addition, there is a pronounced racial gradient in wellbeing among older South Africans. Older Black African adults had significantly lower wellbeing scores than other older adults, which can be traced to the apartheid policies of racialised inequality. Our results also confirmed that marriage, education, and employment all boost personal wellbeing among older adults.

The chapter also examined the effect of a more detailed set of measures relating to social networks, health and healthcare access, and digital technology beliefs and skills on the life satisfaction ratings of older persons. With regards to networking, social isolation and general contact frequency had no significant impact on wellbeing, though face-to-face contact and frequent Internet use positively influenced it. The 2017 health analysis found that self-efficacy and better self-reported health significantly increased life satisfaction, while depressive mood and social strain reduced it. The 2021 analysis similarly identified depression and lack of self-confidence to be inversely associated with life satisfaction among older persons, though these lost significance after accounting for socio-demographic factors. Satisfaction with waiting times and treatment by doctors and nurses positively impacted life satisfaction. Although satisfaction with emergency services initially showed a positive association, this again became non-significant after controlling for socio-demographic factors.

Digital technology seems to have a positive impact on the wellbeing of older adults. As people age, they may find themselves increasingly alone and isolated from others, and unable to participate in social activities. Technology often assists in overcoming some of the barriers that limit social interaction through the use of multiple forms of communication, including text messaging, emails, and audio or video calls (Sen et al., 2021). These mobile devices offer a variety of ways of reaching and communicating with older persons, such as delivering health-related messages as well as providing security or environmental hazard alerts via messaging services (Rademeyer & Maharaj, 2020). Overall, our findings emphasise the positive role of digital skills, frequent Internet use, and engaging in specific Internet activities (especially communication, content creation, and searching for information) on life satisfaction among older persons, with socio-demographic differences playing a role in shaping these relationships. However, the fact that the perceived complexity of the technological turn in society matters for the wellbeing of older citizens also points to a sense of alienation that the digital transition is having on older persons. Those able to access the Internet and who have adapted to digital tools and use it for certain types of activity show that digital technologies can enhance the wellbeing of older persons. Yet those with challenges relating to digital access and capabilities, and who feel alienation and loneliness with the intensification of digital technology in life, tend to exhibit lower wellbeing levels. This raises concern of growing digital inequality among older persons, as well as between older and younger generations.

Ageing in South Africa is occurring in the midst of a great deal of adversity. Widespread poverty, a heavy disease burden, changing household structures, endemic crime, as well as weak or poorly managed governance structures represent significant contextual barriers to the wellbeing of older persons. The ageing of the population has not been a major priority for the national government given the host of problems facing the country. Going forward, more emphasis should be placed on initiatives designed to promote wellbeing across the lifecycle, ensuring that the needs of all individuals are met, regardless of age.

References

Amati, V., Meggiolaro, S., Rivellini, G., & Zaccarin, S. (2018). Social relations and life satisfaction: the role of friends. *Genus, 74*(1), 7.

Baum, F., Musolino, C., Gesesew, H. A., & Popay, J. (2021). New perspective on why women live longer than men: An exploration of power, gender, social determinants, and capitals. *International Journal of Environmental Research and Public Health, 18*(2), 1–23.

Baxter, S., Blank, L., Cantrell, A., & Goyder, E. (2021). Is working in later life good for your health? A systematic review of health outcomes resulting from extended working lives. *BMC Public Health, 21*, 1–11.

Botha, F., & Booysen, F. (2013). The relationship between marital status and life satisfaction among South African adults. *Acta Academica, 45*(2), 150–178.

Cummins, R. A., Eckersley, R., Pallant, J., Van Vugt, J., & Misajon, R. (2003). Developing a national index of subjective wellbeing: The Australian Unity Wellbeing Index. *Social Indicators Research, 64*, 159–190.

Diener, E., & Suh, E. (1997). Measuring quality of life: Economic, social, and subjective indicators. *Social Indicators Research, 40*(1–2), 189–216.

Jivraj, S., Nazroo, J., Vanhoutte, B., & Chandola, T. (2014). Ageing and Subjective Well-Being in Later Life. *The Journals of Gerontology. Series B, Psychological Sciences and Social Sciences, 69*(6), 930–941.

Kollamparambi, U., & Etinzock, M. N. (2019). Subjective well-being impact of old age pension in South Africa: A difference in difference analysis across the gender divide. *South African Journal of Economic and Management Sciences, 22*(1).

Kopylova, N., Greyling, T., & Rossouw, S. (2022). Multidimensional quality of life of older adults in South Africa. *Applied Research in Quality of Life, 17*, 3427–3450.

Maharaj, P., & Roberts, B. (2021). Growing older with dignity: The nature and determinants of quality of life among older people in South Africa. In F. Rojo-Pérez & G. Fernandez-Mayoralas (Eds.), *Active ageing and quality of life: From concepts to applications.* Springer.

Møller, V. (1993). Living with adult children: A benefit assessment of co-resident living arrangements among black and white older South Africans. *Southern African Journal of Gerontology, 2*(1), 10–16.

Møller, V., & Ferreira, M. (1992). Successful ageing in South Africa: opportunity structures and subjective wellbeing. *Southern African Journal of Gerontology, 1*(1), 5–8.

Moore, E. (2024). *Older persons, care needs & social grants in South Africa.* University of Cape Town.

Ntozini, A., & Abdullahi, A. A. (2021). Loneliness and psychological well-being among the elderly in Buffalo City, South Africa. *Journal of Psychology in Africa, 31*(4), 383–389.

Patterson, S. E., & Margolis, R. (2023). Family ties and older adult well-being: Incorporating social networks and proximity. *The Journals of Gerontology. Series B, Psychological Sciences and Social Sciences, 78*(12), 2080–2089.

Peltzer, K., & Phaswana-Mafuya, N. (2013). Depression and associated factors in older adults in South Africa. *Global Health Action, 6*, 1–9.

Phaswana-Mafuya, N., & Peltzer, K. (2017). Prevalence of loneliness and associated factors among older adults in South Africa. *Global Journal of Health Science, 9*(12), 1–8.

Putrik, P., van Amelsvoort, L., Mujakovic, S., Kunst, A. E., van Oers, H., Kant, I., Jansen, M. W., & De Vries, N. K. (2019). Assessing the role of criminality in neighbourhood safety feelings and self-reported health: results from a cross-sectional study in a Dutch municipality. *BMC Public Health, 19*, 920.

Rademeyer, S., & Maharaj, P. (2020). Patterns and trends. In P. Maharaj (Ed.), *Health and care in old age in Africa.* Routledge.

Ralston, M. (2018). The role of older persons' environment in ageing well: Quality of life, illness, and community context in South Africa. *Gerontologist, 58*(1), 111–120.

Reich, A. J., Claunch, K. D., Verdeja, M. A., Dungan, M. T., Anderson, S., Clayton, C. K., Goates, M. C., & Thacker, E. L. (2020). What does "successful ageing" mean to you? - systematic review and cross-cultural comparison of lay perspectives of older adults in 13 countries, 2010–2020. *Journal of Cross-Cultural Gerontology, 35*(4), 455–447.

Riumallo-Herl, C., Canning, D., & Kabudula, C. (2019). Health inequalities in the South African elderly: The importance of the measure of social-economic status. *The Journal of the Economics of Ageing, 14*, 100191.

Rodriguez-Blazquez, C., Frades-Payo, B., Forjaz, M. J., Ayala, A., Martinez-Martin, P., Fernandez-Mayoralas, G., & Rojo-Perez, F. (2011). Psychometric properties of the International Wellbeing Index in community dwellings older adults. *International Psychogeriatrics, 23*(1), 161–169.

Schatz, E., Gomez-Olive, X., Ralston, M., Menken, J., & Tollman, S. (2012). The impact of pensions on health and wellbeing in rural South Africa: Does gender matter? *Social Science and Medicine, 75*(10), 1864–1873.

Sen, K., Prybutok, G., & Prybutok, V. (2021). The use of digital technology for social wellbeing reduces social isolation in older adults: A systematic review. *Population Health, 17*, 101020.

Statistics South Africa. (2023). *The social profile of older persons, 2017–2021*. Statistics South Africa.

Voukelatou, V., Gabrielli, L., Miliou, J., Cresci, S., Sharma, R., Tesconi, M., & Pappalardo, L. (2019). Measuring objective and subjective well-being: Dimensions and data. *International Journal of Data Science and Analytics, 11*, 279–309.

Wadsworth, T. (2016). Marriage and subjective well-being. *Social Indicators Research, 126*(3), 1025–1048.

Walsh, K., Scharf, T., & Keating, N. (2017). Social exclusion of older persons: A scoping review and conceptual framework. *European Journal of Ageing, 14*(1), 81–98.

4

Poverty Among Older People in South Africa

Shanaaz Dunn and Pranitha Maharaj

Abstract South Africa has one of the most rapidly ageing populations in Africa, and the proportion of older persons has been increasing steadily over time. While living longer is a significant achievement, it is equally concerning as ageing is occurring in a context where poverty is widespread. This study uses data from the 2017 South African National Income Dynamics Survey to explore poverty among older people. The study examines key socio-demographic and economic determinants of poverty among older people in South Africa. The results indicate that more older people are living below the upper-bound poverty line in comparison to those who are food poor. Older Black African women with

S. Dunn (✉)
Developmental, Capable and Ethical State, Human Sciences Research Council, Durban, South Africa
e-mail: SDunn@hsrc.ac.za

P. Maharaj
School of Built Environment and Development Studies, University of KwaZulu-Natal, Durban, South Africa
e-mail: Maharajp7@ukzn.ac.za

P. Maharaj (ed.), *Navigating Ageing in South Africa*, Sustainable Development Goals Series, https://doi.org/10.1007/978-981-97-9088-3_4

lower levels of education who have never been married, have a higher risk of living in poverty. More older people accessing a grant live in poverty. This demonstrates the importance of social protection in alleviating household poverty.

Keywords Poverty • Older people • NIDS • Estimates • South Africa

Introduction

The African continent is one of the poorest in the world, suffering from the effects of multi-dimensional poverty. It has the highest percentage of people living below the poverty line of less than US$1.90 per day (UNDP, 2018). Increasingly, there is widespread concern that older people are ageing in the context of high levels of poverty. As of 2019, in Sub-Saharan Africa, approximately 3% of the population were 65 years or older and this is projected to increase to 13% by 2100 (UNDESA, 2019a). An increase in life expectancy is a remarkable gain yet many nations are not well prepared to deal with the challenges, which includes old age dependency and poverty among the elderly. Therefore, tackling poverty among the elderly should be prioritised because it enables people to experience a better quality of life (Patsios, 2006).

There have been nation-wide efforts in developing countries to eradicate poverty; however, despite these efforts poverty still remains a major challenge (Lilenstein et al., 2016; UNDP, 2018; World Bank, 2015). In many of the lesser developed countries and those that rank low on the Human Development Index (HDI), many of which are within Africa, there are still high levels of malnutrition, low levels of water and sanitation provision, and prominent health concerns (UNDP, 2018). Even though there have been observable achievements in economic growth, the sub-Saharan African region is characterised by extreme socio-economic deprivation and harsh living conditions (Niño-Zarazúa et al., 2012; Sembene, 2015; UNDP, 2018).

Ageing presents an additional risk of becoming or remaining poor (UNDESA, 2015b). South Africa has one of the most rapidly ageing populations in Africa and the proportion of persons aged 60 years and older has been increasing steadily over time (UNDESA, 2019b). There are more than 5 million people aged 60 years and older in the population, equating to 9.2% of the total share of the overall population (Statistics South Africa, 2022). In general, the number of older persons increased across all provinces, with Gauteng and KwaZulu-Natal having the highest number of the older population (Statistics South Africa, 2022). The phenomenon of population ageing has become more significant in the South African context, especially during recent decades, as those aged 60 years and older are increasing noticeably, in both percentage and number. Living longer is a significant achievement; however, this is concerning as ageing is occurring in a context where poverty is widespread (Statistics South Africa, 2011, 2018b; UNDP, 2018).

As people age they become more vulnerable and are more likely to experience economic insecurity and poverty (Braimah & Rosenberg, 2021). Estimates suggest that despite the general decline in poverty between 2006 and 2011, poverty levels in South Africa rose in 2015 (Statistics South Africa, 2017a). This translates into over 30.4 million South Africans living in poverty in 2015 (Statistics South Africa, 2017b). South Africa has a medium HDI and ranks 114 out of 189 countries (UNDP, 2022). A significant proportion (83%) of the population are living in households with access to improved sanitation facilities (UNDP, 2022). This indicates that there still is a need to improve the living conditions as well as accessibility of basic services for many. As a result, there is widespread concern that people are ageing in South Africa in the context of high levels of poverty. High levels of poverty, coupled with a growing ageing population, highlights the importance of addressing quality of life at older ages. The focus of this chapter is on profiling poverty among older people.

Social Security as a Safety Net for South Africans

Ageing can influence a household's economic well-being because it has an influence on employment (Riumallo-Herl et al., 2019). A South African study conducted by Riumallo-Herl et al. (2019) reveals that employment rates start to decline before people reach retirement age which is usually around the age of 60 years. This means that a large share of older people who are considered economically active are not participating in the labour force. Unemployment directly and indirectly affects older people as being out of the labour force is strongly associated with lower income and thus a lower capacity to provide any financial support (Riumallo-Herl et al., 2019). Older people are also affected by the unemployment of a child or relative. With limited means to provide support, children are no longer financially capable of supporting elderly parents. In much of Africa, the traditional safety net for the elderly is the extended family (Aboderin, 2017); however, this support system is severely compromised especially when adult children are too poor to support parents and are burdened with the effects of high levels of unemployment (Tanga et al., 2019). As a result, many older people become the primary breadwinners and caregivers of their families (Kalomo & Besthorn, 2018). In the past, children and grandchildren were the primary providers and caregivers of elderly family members (Aboderin, 2017). However, changing patterns of urbanisation and globalisation have exposed older people to the risk of poverty with very little care and support (Aboderin, 2017; Randel, 2017).

Older people have limited capacity to engage in the formal workforce due to their declining physical capability. This places them at an elevated risk of poverty and as a consequence they experience poor health, food insecurity, and lack of access to basic necessities (Pirrie et al., 2020). A South African study found that older people felt overlooked in primary healthcare provision and had very little trust in the system (Kelly et al., 2019). Another study in South Africa suggests improved health service utilisation among those who access a pension (Lloyd-Sherlock & Agrawal, 2014). South Africa has a unique old age grant or pension system which is not available in most other African countries. This social support system is instrumental in ensuring improved health and wellbeing of older people. A study conducted by Etinzock and Kollamparambil (2019) suggests that female recipients have a positive and significant change in well-being because they are able to access the old age grant. Female headed households are associated with higher levels of poverty than male headed households (Nwosu & Ndinda, 2018). A study by Schatz and Madhavan (2011) suggests that a significant percentage of women aged 60 years and older are heads of households and this percentage has increased from 2000 (10%) to 2005 (12%). This percentage is higher than that of older men for both time periods (Schatz & Madhavan, 2011). Changing household structures results in more older women assuming headship which highlights the importance of government provision of social support for the elderly (Beard & Bloom, 2015).

South Africa is a middle-income country and has the largest portion of older people in the Southern region of Africa. It is imperative to focus on South Africa because literature on poverty and old age is dated. Additionally, past policies during the apartheid era have left a legacy of inequality, exclusion, and poverty that persists (World Bank, 2018). The potential implications of poverty in older age highlights the need for more research to be generated in this field in order to make recommendations that will enable policy to be geared towards accommodating the requirements of the rapidly ageing population. Older people play significant contributory roles in their families, especially in Africa. However, poverty and social exclusion represent two of the most significant barriers for older people (Kwan & Walsh, 2018). Providing empirical evidence on old age poverty is critical to fully actualise the opportunities and address key challenges of population ageing. In South Africa, ensuring the well-being of older people during this time is of paramount importance, given the experience of ageing and poverty within the country.

A better understanding of the discourse of old age poverty is required in the context of global ageing. In the development discourse, eradication of poverty is a key priority for policy makers worldwide. The Sustainable Development Goals (SDGs) iterates that poverty eradication is the greatest global challenge facing the world today and the central focus is to end poverty in all its forms. However, there is limited focus on old age poverty (Kwan & Walsh, 2018). The purpose of this research is to shed insight into old age poverty by examining key socio-demographic and economic determinants such as age, gender, and marital and employment status among others. Understanding poverty in later life is important for developing appropriate policy because of the valuable contribution of older people. Focusing on people aged 60 years and older, this study explores how poverty varies across South Africa's ageing population.

Methodology

This research uses the National Incomes and Dynamics Survey (NIDS) for the analysis. NIDS is a panel study with a nationally representative sample of over 28,000 individuals in 7300 households across the country. The survey has since 2008 been repeated with the same household members every 2 years. The survey collected information on changes in poverty and wellbeing; household composition and structure; fertility and mortality; migration; labour market participation and economic activity; and health and education (SALDRU, 2019). For this research, NIDS wave five, conducted in 2017, is used with the specific intention to explore poverty across the ageing South African population. The analysis extends across three poverty lines for robustness of the estimates and to highlight any significant outliers and patterns; however, the focus of the study is on the food poverty line. Since 2020, the COVID-19 pandemic has accelerated food insecurity across the world and those who are vulnerable, particularly older people, have been adversely affected. Therefore, even though the data does not reflect estimates from the current pandemic it does shed insight about the existing experience of poverty among older people and outlines and highlights the imminent need for reliable social safety as well as sustainable systems to accommodate the older population.

Poverty can be measured either objectively or subjectively. For the purpose of this research, the analysis includes the objective measurement of poverty. This is the most appropriate measure for a study of this nature as objective poverty can be captured quantitatively. Objective poverty can be measured using either an absolute or relative approach. This research uses both approaches to obtain a holistic view of the estimates pertaining to poverty at older ages. The absolute approach refers to a poverty line which is based on the minimum income needed to afford essential items, like enough food to meet a daily calorie requirement (Haughton & Khandker, 2009; Statistics South Africa, 2019). Relative poverty helps to identify the poorest sector of the population by setting a poverty line at a specific percentage of the average or middle income per person (Govendor et al., 2006). In South Africa, there have been many studies focused on money-metric poverty from a range of datasets; however, very few use a holistic approach and produce research with all measures, hence this research aims to bridge that gap (Leibbrandt et al., 2006; Rogan, 2018).

Variables and Measures

This study specifically focuses on people aged 60 years and older. In addition, for this study, the key outcome (dependent) variable is poverty; either an older person is poor or non-poor based on the condition of the poverty line constructed. The explanatory variables of interest for this study included age, gender, race, education, marital status, employment status, and access to an old age grant. Most of these variables were coded into binomial categories. Age was restricted to those individuals aged 60 years and older. This condition was selected on the general consensus in the literature that defines an older person. The age of 60 or 65, roughly equivalent to retirement ages in most developed countries, is said to be the beginning of old age (Gorman, 2000). Additionally, in the South African context any person who is 60 years and older is eligible for an old age grant. The race variable was binary coded to capture Black African South Africans, and 'Other' which included Indians, Coloureds, and Whites. These categories were based on Statistics South Africa's classifications (Statistics South Africa, 2018a).

Poverty Lines

The three key dependent variables for this study were upper, lower, and food poverty lines. The construction of the poverty lines is based on the total household expenditure relative to the total household size or members per household and then further segregated by the monetary value of the defined poverty thresholds. According to Statistics South Africa (2018b), poverty lines are important tools that allow for the statistical reporting of poverty levels and patterns, as well as the planning, monitoring, and evaluation of poverty reduction programmes and policies. In essence, it is a set of cut-off points which separate the poor from the non-poor. This research specifically examines food, lower, and upper poverty lines. The food poverty line is based on the daily calories a person needs to survive. The lower and upper bound poverty lines both include non-food items. However, with regard to the lower bound poverty line a person would need to sacrifice food items to acquire non-food items; however, with regard to the upper bound poverty line, people are able to purchase both adequate food and non-food items (Statistics South Africa, 2018b).

The poverty lines for this research analysis were constructed based on data provided by Statistics South Africa (2018b). For the analysis, poverty lines were constructed based on the inflated adjusted national poverty lines provided for April 2017 prices (in South African Rands). These prices are based on the estimates linked to the values for March in that year. The food poverty line was R531 in April 2017 per person per month. This refers to the amount of money that an individual will need to afford the minimum required daily energy intake. The lower bound poverty line was R758 in April 2017 per person per month. This refers to the food poverty line plus the average amount derived from non-food items of households whose total expenditure is equal to the food poverty line. The upper bound poverty line was R1 138 in April 2017 per person per month. This refers to the food poverty line plus the average amount derived from non-food items of households whose food expenditure is equal to the food poverty line. This translates into less than US$1.90 a day. The use of the three different poverty lines allows for comparisons between varying socio-demographic characteristics. Poverty can be measured at the individual or household level. This research measures poverty at the household level; however, disaggregates the analysis and output by varying individual characteristics (age and gender) of those who live in households below the poverty lines. Exploring the experience of poverty of households, in which an older person is a resident, is an important step towards understanding their quality of life.

Analytical Approach

The data was analysed using STATA version 15. In the analysis, design weights were applied to the data. The use of design weights allows for the correction of non-response as well as provides unbiased estimates of the population defined by the sampling rules. Weights are used to make inferences about the population from the sample by adjusting for unequal probabilities of selection and for non-response. The complex survey design and sampling weights were also considered to adjust for representativeness of the estimates.

Descriptive statistics were calculated to determine the characteristics of the study sample. To investigate the statistical association between poverty and older people and other explanatory variables, a multivariate analysis was conducted to reveal causality in the results. Logistic regression was used to explore the determinants that are associated with poverty at older ages. The analysis was restricted to those who are 60 years and older. This condition was defined to ensure that the results are relevant to the older population under investigation. Various models (unadjusted and adjusted linear models) were constructed using dependent variables of the food, upper bound, and lower bound poverty line. The main difference between the unadjusted and adjusted odds ratios is the addition of variables in the adjusted model. In the unadjusted model, each independent variable was entered into the model individually, while the adjusted included all variables. Both unadjusted and adjusted odds ratios (OR) are presented along with the 95% confidence intervals (CI) and the corresponding p-values to denote the statistical significance of the OR. Estimates were considered statistically significant at $p < 0.05$.

Results

Descriptive Statistics

The estimates are broadly categorised into aggregated estimates and thereafter focused on individual level characteristics of the study sample. The estimates suggest that the average household size is 5.57, which was calculated by averaging the household size variable. The average monthly income for each household is estimated at R9069.75, which was calculated by averaging the total monthly income per household. The average household per capita, which was calculated by dividing the average monthly income by the average household size, is estimated at R1868.76.

Estimates from the adult data file indicate that 1833 individuals are below the age of 18 years. The majority of the study sample are aged 18–59 years (N=18,509) whereas those who are 60 years and older constitute a smaller number (N=3545). Estimates pertaining to poverty displayed in Table 4.1 suggest that a considerable percentage of older people live in poorer households, which ranges from 12% to 14%. Most older people who live in households below the defined poverty lines have good to fair health status with very few reporting excellent health. Estimates pertaining to household structure, as evidenced in Table 4.1 indicate that most older people are married and live with their partners. When asked if they lived with their children, the majority of older people who live in a household below the defined poverty line indicated that they reside with their biological children.

Study Sample Characteristics

The study sample for NIDS wave 5 consists of 3545 people aged 60 years and older. For representivity and generalisability, weighted percentages are displayed in Table 4.2. In 2017, the majority of older people (59.31%) were between the ages of 60 and 69 years whereas only 11.17% were 80 years and older. A large percentage of older people were Black African (72.58%) and female (66.57%). Education differentials indicate that the majority had no schooling or a primary level education (65.87%) with a

Table 4.1 Aggregate poverty estimates, wave five (2017)

	Food poverty line N (%)	Lower bound poverty line N (%)	Upper bound poverty line N (%)
Broad age categories			
Under 18 years	792 (10.60)	1076 (9.90)	1351 (9.30)
18–59 years	5704 (76.60)	8251 (76.20)	10,999 (76.10)
60 years and above	1833 (12.70)	1505 (13.90)	2112 (14.60)
Total	**7442 (100.00)**	**10,832 (100.00)**	**14,462 (100.00)**
Health status of elderly			
Excellent	87 (9.20)	110 (7.30)	150 (7.10)
Very good	184 (19.50)	290 (19.30)	411 (19.50)
Good	368 (38.90)	592 (39.30)	798 (37.80)
Fair	228 (24.10)	380 (25.20)	559 (26.50)
Poor	79 (8.40)	133 (8.80)	193 (9.10)
Total	**946 (100.00)**	**1505 (100.00)**	**2111 (100.00)**
Living arrangements of elderly			
Married and living with partner only	307 (89.50)	508 (88.50)	749 (89.00)
Unmarried and cohabiting	35 (10.20)	63 (11.00)	80 (9.60)
Not living with partner	1 (0.30)	3 (0.50)	5 (0.60)
Total	**343 (100.00)**	**574 (100.00)**	**834 (100.00)**
Living arrangements			
Living with biological children only	456 (67.60)	673 (64.20)	874 (60.80)
Not living with biological children	219 (32.40)	376 (35.80)	563 (39.20)
Total	**675 (100.00)**	**1049 (100.00)**	**1437 (100.00)**

Source: Calculation from NIDS wave five

smaller percentage with secondary level education or higher (34.13%). The majority were also unmarried (54.42%). Further estimates reveal that 84.79% of older people were at that time unemployed. Additionally, the majority of older people (77.60%) were recipients of an old age grant. These estimates are displayed in Table 4.2.

Table 4.3 specifically focuses on the population aged 60 years and older who were categorised according to the food poverty line as well as the lower and upper bound poverty lines. Results indicated that this percentage is highest for those that live below the upper bound poverty line (59.60%) and lower for those who are food poor (26.70%). Segregated

Table 4.2 Socio-demographics characteristics of the study sample aged 60 years and older—wave five, 2017 (N=3545)

Characteristic	N	%
Age		
60–69	2103	59.31
70–79	1047	29.53
80+	396	11.17
Sex		
Females	2360	66.57
Males	1185	33.43
Race		
Black African	2572	72.58
Other	972	27.43
Education		
No schooling or primary	2326	65.87
Secondary or higher	1205	34.13
Marital status		
Married	1615	45.58
Unmarried/other	1928	54.42
Employment status		
Unemployed	3004	84.79
Employed	539	15.21
Old age grant recipient		
Yes	2751	77.60
No	764	22.40

Source: Calculation from NIDS wave five

by race and gender, the majority of those aged 60 years and older who live in households that experience poverty are Black African and female. In addition, a higher percentage of individuals aged 60 years and older who have no schooling or a primary level education live in households that are categorised as either food poor or below the upper and lower bound poverty lines. Table 4.3 suggests that there is a considerable number of individuals aged 60 years and older that are currently unemployed and live below the defined poverty lines. Even though the majority of the study population accessed an old age grant, a large percentage remained below the food poverty line (90.60%), lower bound poverty line (90.80%), and upper bound poverty line (90.20%).

Table 4.3 Socio-demographic characteristics of the study sample aged 60 and older in poverty—wave five (2017)

	Lower bound poverty line N (%)	Upper bound poverty line N (%)	Food poverty line N (%)
Poor/non-poor status			
Not poor	2040 (57.50)	1433 (40.40)	2599 (73.30)
Poor	1505 (42.50)	2112 (59.60)	946 (26.70)
Sex			
Females	1075 (71.40)	1471 (69.60)	689 (72.80)
Males	430 (28.60)	641 (30.40)	257 (27.20)
Race			
Black African	1378 (91.60)	1875 (88.80)	875 (92.50)
Other	127 (8.40)	237 (11.20)	71 (7.50)
Education			
No schooling or primary	1314 (87.60)	1766 (83.80)	854 (90.60)
Secondary or higher	186 (12.40)	341 (16.20)	89 (9.40)
Marital status			
Married	577 (38.30)	843 (39.90)	348 (36.80)
Unmarried/other	928 (61.70)	1269 (60.10)	598 (63.20)
Employment status			
Unemployed	1355 (90.10)	1878 (89.00)	854 (90.30)
Employed	149 (9.90)	233 (11.00)	92 (9.70)
Old age grant recipient			
Yes	1367 (90.80)	1905 (90.20)	857 (90.60)
No	138 (9.20)	207 (9.80)	89 (9.40)

Source: Calculation from NIDS wave five

Regression Analysis

Table 4.4 presents the results from the multivariate logistic regression to determine the socio demographic and economic factors that are associated with the experience of poverty among the older population. The odds ratio is presented with the significance and confidence intervals. The table presents both the unadjusted and adjusted odds ratio. The main difference between the unadjusted and adjusted odds ratio is the addition of variables in the adjusted model. The adjusted model holds all other independent variables in a model constant. The unadjusted odds for

Table 4.4 Determinants of old age poverty using a logistic regression, wave five (2017)

		Lower bound poverty line		Upper bound poverty line		Food poverty line	
		Unadjusted	Adjusted	Unadjusted	Adjusted	Unadjusted	Adjusted
		OR [95% CI]		OR [95% CI]		OR [95% CI]	
Race	Black African	1.00	1.00	1.00	1.00	1.00	1.00
	Other	0.1302*** [0.1064–0.1593]	0.2134*** [0.1722–0.2645]	0.1198*** [0.1010–0.1421]	0.1946*** [0.1717–0.2341]	0.1528*** [0.1184–0.1972]	0.2598*** [0.1986–0.3398]
Gender	Male	1.00	1.00	1.00	1.00	1.00	1.00
	Female	1.4688*** [1.2725–1.6954]	1.1710 [0.9792–1.4003]	1.4042*** [1.2191–1.6175]	1.0817 [0.8769–1.3034]	1.4887*** [1.2634–1.7545]	1.1998 [0.9886–1.4561]
Level of education	None or primary	1.00	1.00	1.00	1.00	1.00	1.00
	Secondary or higher	0.1405*** [0.1178–0.1677]	0.2191*** [0.1816–0.2642]	0.1251*** [0.1069–0.1464]	0.1956*** [0.1649–0.2321]	0.1374*** [0.1090–0.1733]	0.2048*** [0.1637–0.2653]
Marital status	Married	1.00	1.00	1.00	1.00	1.00	1.00
	Unmarried/ Other	1.4578*** [1.2731–1.6693]	0.9840 [0.8308–1.1654]	1.4536*** [1.2696–1.6643]	0.9315 [0.7791–1.1137]	1.47*** [1.2627–1.7148]	1.03 [0.8672–1.2445]
Employment status	Unemployed	1.00	1.00	1.00	1.00	1.00	1.00
	Employed	0.4649*** [0.3799–0.5690]	0.6560*** [0.5215–0.8253]	0.4565*** [0.3791–0.5497]	0.6479*** [0.5176–0.8109]		0.7456* [0.5773–0.9679]
N			3526		3526		3526
Log likelihood			-1980.7212		-1829.9024		-1777.4921
Chi2			0.0000		0.0000		0.0000

Significant at ***p<0.001 **p<0.01 *p<0.05
Source: Calculation from NIDS wave five

those aged 60 years and older who lived in households that were below the lower bound poverty line indicate that other racial groups were 87% less likely than Black Africans to live in households below the lower bound poverty line. The same outcome was observed in the adjusted model, where 79% of other racial groups were less likely than Black Africans to live in households below the lower bound poverty line and the association was highly significant. Similar outcomes were observed for the adjusted estimates for other racial groups who lived in households below the upper bound (79% less likely than Black Africans to live below the upper bound poverty line) and food poverty line (75% less likely than Black Africans to live below the food poverty line).

The gender covariate revealed that women have significantly higher odds of living in a household below the defined poverty lines. In all the unadjusted models, women are over 40% more likely to live within households below the upper and lower bound and food poverty line. These associations were highly significant. However, in the adjusted model, gender did not have a significant effect on the outcome. A higher education attainment is associated with a lower likelihood of an elderly person living in a household below the defined poverty lines. All results were highly significant at the confidence intervals. The marital status covariate yielded varying results across the adjusted and unadjusted models. In the unadjusted models those that were married were less likely to live in a household that was below the defined poverty lines whereas those that were unmarried were more likely to live in a household below the defined poverty lines. However, there was no significant association in the adjusted models for those that were 60 years and older, unmarried and lived in households below the food poverty line. Employment status had a significant effect on those who were 60 years and older and lived in households below the defined poverty lines. Both the unadjusted and adjusted models suggest that those who are 60 years and older and are currently employed are less likely to live in households below the defined poverty lines and these associations were all significant.

Factors Associated with Old Age Poverty

This study examines key socio-demographic and economic determinants of poverty among older people in South Africa. The findings of this study raise widespread concern for the need for effective and sufficient measures in place to alleviate the burden associated with ageing at the individual, the family, and the government level. This is especially concerning in the South African context because the experience of poverty is nuanced among the very young and very old segments of the population (Statistics South Africa, 2017a). The estimates from the study suggest that a large number of people live in households below the defined poverty lines. This is concerning because it suggests that the South African National Development Plan (NDP) 2030 is not likely to be achieved. The NDP is a nation-wide plan to effectively eliminate poverty and reduce inequality by 2030. The NDP 2030 proposes to reduce the proportion of all people living below the lower bound poverty line by 2030 (Statistics South Africa, 2017b). Thus outlining the importance of government-funded grant systems. According to Statistics South Africa (2017a), there was a general decline in poverty between 2006 and 2011; however, a closer look at the upper-bound poverty line indicated that one out of every two South Africans were poor in 2015. For this period, the poverty headcount increased to 55.5% (approximately 30.4 million people) from 53.2% in 2011. These findings corroborate with the findings from this study which indicate that there were more older people currently living within households below the defined poverty lines.

In many countries, the absence of social protection systems, especially for older people, contributes greatly to food and income insecurity. Older people are particularly vulnerable to economic insecurity as well as poverty, with limited options available (UNDESA, 2015a). A fairly large portion of the study population aged 60 years and older accessed the old age grant. Access to an old age grant has a significant effect on the experience of poverty in a household. The old age grant assists in sustaining the household and offsets the experience of being food poor. This is evident when grant systems in many countries fail to meet the needs of those for whom it is provided (UNDESA, 2015a). Older people are more likely to live in households that experience poverty. This is expected because the old age grant is meant for individuals who cannot afford to support themselves financially and have an income or asset valued above a certain threshold (South African Government, 2020). For practical implications on a nation-wide and continental scale, it is suggested that broader efforts emerge to address poverty among the elderly especially in contexts with a rapidly growing older population. If poverty among older people is left unchecked, other social and economic factors will be adversely impacted.

A key factor of older people's poverty is their reduced capacity to work which results in their lack of income (Heslop & Gorman, 2002). As a result, it becomes difficult to sustain a healthy lifestyle and access healthcare because of affordability. This means that many older people are left vulnerable and are further exposed to the challenges that are exacerbated by poverty (Smeeding & Sandstrom, 2005). Getting old presents a significant, additional risk of becoming and/or remaining poor. Results from this study reveal that a large percentage of older people are currently unemployed, within both the time periods, and this is expected given their limited capacity to perform tasks. Many older people are often part of the informal trading sector, whereby small-scale goods are sold, and they risk being overlooked by broader economic efforts. This, in essence, will exacerbate the experience of poverty among the aged. In addition to this, the biological effect of ageing leads to a gradual decrease in physical and mental capacity and a growing risk of contracting illnesses and age-related diseases. As a result, older people are likely to experience difficulty in physical activity and are less likely to work or be involved in income generating activities (WHO, 2015). Results from this study indicate that earning an income through employment significantly offsets the experience of poverty within a household. However, household poverty of older people was not significantly affected by employment status when other covariates were in place. Many older people rely on the informal economy for their livelihoods (Statistics South Africa, 2011) and results from the study reveal that a large percentage of older people are currently unemployed, and this is expected given their limited capacity to perform tasks. This will exacerbate the experience of poverty among the elderly. This highlights the need for stronger social security systems, not just in South Africa, but across the continent as a means of offsetting the experience of poverty. Further to this, results from this study indicate that earning an income through employment significantly offsets the experience of poverty in a household.

Improvement in education over time is an indicator of development (Statistics South Africa, 2011). Educational attainment among older people is generally low, with a smaller percentage of people having attained a secondary or higher education in comparison to those with none or a lower level of education, as evidenced from this study. In South Africa older people have a lower level of education; however, there have been improvements across time (Statistics South Africa, 2011). The state of education among older people can be largely attributed to the historical context where Black South Africans were afforded very little opportunity to pursue an education during the apartheid era. Hence, the adverse implications of a non-coherent education policy, which was largely based on race (Morris & Hyslop, 1991), had long-lasting implications for the country which took decades to redress. According to Statistics South Africa (2011) the proportion of older people with no schooling has decreased from 47% in 1996 to 28% in 2011. The prevalence of poverty among the elderly has been linked to low levels of literacy. Some studies reference educational attainment as an important determinant of socioeconomic status (Darin-Mattsson et al., 2017). Therefore, increasing access to educational attainment will offset the effects of lower socioeconomic status.

Poverty rates among older women are highest among those who are not married, as evidenced from this study and existing literature (Lin et al., 2017). Estimates suggest that the prevalence will rise significantly over the next decades (Smeeding & Sandstrom, 2005). This is expected as a vast amount of literature documents the feminisation of poverty, which suggests that an increasing percentage of the world's poor are women (McLanahan & Kelly, 2006; Moghadam, 2005). Torres (2014) observed that women continue to face significant economic disadvantage in old age, and the proportion of older women in poverty increases as women age. Results from this study indicate that older women are at much greater risk of experiencing poverty in comparison to older men. This corroborates with the findings of other studies (Smeeding & Sandstrom, 2005; Torres, 2014). Poverty among older women is usually a result of various factors including their lower labour force participation and the fact that they often have shorter and interrupted careers due to childbearing and rearing. The United Nations (UNDESA, 2015b) suggests that in the sub-Saharan African context, households headed by older women are more prone to poverty than households headed by older men, especially in parts of the region that are patriarchal. South Africa also has a legacy of apartheid which meant that Black African women were not given the opportunity to engage in formal paid employment. It was usually the responsibility of men to migrate for salaried employment while women stayed home and maintained the homestead (Walker, 1990). Older women living alone or in one-person households are more likely than men to be living in poverty (UNDESA, 2015a). In this context, women have more access to opportunities; however, poverty persists for older women because they experience a lifetime of unpaid work which is sometimes interrupted by childcare responsibilities, divorce, labour market discrimination, and inequality. Not surprising then women are often subjected to poverty later in life (Torres, 2014). Thus, the findings of this study have important implications for improving the quality of life of older people. Timely estimates are needed to redirect and prioritise efforts to minimise the effects of poverty experienced by older people.

The novelty of this study lies in the contribution that it makes towards knowledge about poverty and ageing in South Africa by specifically drawing on the NIDS datasets which has been under-utilised as a source of information. With a clear understanding of poverty and ageing, governments can make informed decisions about the challenges that will affect the population that are most vulnerable. Drawing on the global pandemic of SARS-CoV-2, it is clear that the long-term increase in inequalities and neglect of public services have weakened the ability of societies to deal with external, sudden shocks. This has further exacerbated current challenges which are proving to be difficult to address, such as poverty and access to quality healthcare. Those without secure employment and lack of social protection are severely affected by the impact of the virus (Clark, 2020).

To ensure health and overall well-being for everyone, poverty eradication efforts and strategies needs to be geared towards those experiencing the greatest burdens. Poverty is an important, universal human challenge that affects people of all ages. To ensure credible and effective action in addressing poverty and inequality, information on the poverty situation is required on a regular basis. Information on the changing trends of the experience of poverty among the older population is key to evidence-based decision-making which can enable poverty reduction strategies that is geared towards the ageing population. This will enable a nation-wide attempt to ensure good health and wellbeing for the ageing population (Statistics South Africa, 2008). The findings also highlight specific characteristics of old age poverty, outlining the way forward in terms of redress and equality especially among the segment of the population where poverty is most profound. Additionally, this can enable a global effort towards the reduction of poverty at older ages, as well as enable other researchers and initiatives to segregate their analysis to capture the heterogeneity (or uniqueness) of their population. The risk of old age poverty is generally more pronounced in less developed countries where social protection coverage is inadequate or absent, and where many older persons rely only on family support. This implies the need for reinforced policy interventions, primarily through social protection. Public social security pensions are important solutions to ensure income security. Public social security pensions have become essential tools to ensure that older persons receive a stable income after the end of their working life and throughout their old age. Satumba et al. (2017) suggest that social grants are well-targeted and have significantly reduced poverty levels in areas with high poverty rates in diverse geographic locations in South Africa, among the African population, in female-headed households, and in rural areas. In South Africa there are social wage interventions and other initiatives such as the Indigent Support Programme which is the provision of free basic services to those who cannot afford to pay; however, many older persons continue to live without adequate social protection coverage (UNDESA, 2015b).

Given the quantitative focus of this study, it is not without limitations. The primary limitation of this study is that cross-sectional analysis is performed on a panel study. Although this study does provide insights about poverty and ageing it does not consider the factors which cause an individual to transition in and out of poverty. This can only be gathered from a panel analysis where the complexity of human behaviour will allow for further examination. Additionally, panel analysis allows for greater variability and greater control of endogeneity. The researchers did not perform a panel analysis and as a result there was no control for endogeneity. To compensate for this limitation, the researchers acknowledge that population heterogeneity is an important factor to consider, especially in the South African context, given the diversified characteristics of the population. Therefore, the causal inferential analysis is conducted at a group level which clearly defines the population under interest. Another limitation of this study is that there was no analysis of the poverty gap and severity. The poverty gap provides the minimum cost of eliminating poverty if transfers are specifically targeted. This measure does not reflect changes in inequality among the poor which is an important factor in the South African context that could be explored in detail in future research. In addition, future research should focus on provincial variations in poverty among older people in South Africa.

Conclusion

This study uses national data from South Africa to examine sociodemographic and economic determinants of poverty among older people who are often less economically active and are often overlooked in empirical research. Older people are important members in society and they play key roles in their families. They provide care for sick family members and their children and use their old age grant to financially support their households. Poverty among older people in South Africa needs to be strategically addressed to alleviate the burden. Hence, there should be greater efforts to improve the health and overall well-being of older people. This is a step towards poverty eradication among this vulnerable sector of the population. Based on the findings of the study, it is recommended that the existing social security systems for older people are strengthened. Further to this, the government can also implement long-term, sustainable health and care provisions for older people to ensure better health outcomes and an improved quality of life.

References

Aboderin, I. (2017). *Intergenerational support and old age in Africa*. Routledge.

Beard, H., & Bloom, D. E. (2015). Towards a comprehensive public health response to population ageing. *Lancet, 385*(9968), 658–661.

Braimah, J. A., & Rosenberg, M. W. (2021). "They do not care about us anymore": Understanding the situation of older people in Ghana. *International Journal of Environmental Research and Public Health, 18*(5), 2337.

Clark, G. (2020). COVID-19: Remaking the social contract. *The Lancet, 395*(10234), 1401.

Darin-Mattsson, A., Fors, S., & Kåreholt, I. (2017). Different indicators of socioeconomic status and their relative importance as determinants of health in old age. *International Journal for Equity in Health, 16*(1), 1–11.

Etinzock, M. N., & Kollamparambil, U. (2019). Subjective well-being impact of old age pension in South Africa: A difference in difference analysis across the gender divide. *South African Journal of Economic and Management Sciences, 22*(1), 1–12.

Gorman, M. (2000). Development and the rights of older people. In J. Randel, T. German, & D. Ewing (Eds.), *The ageing and development report: Poverty, independence and the world's older people*. Earthscan Publications Ltd.

Govendor, P., Kambaran, N., Patchett, N., Ruddle, A., Torr, G., & Van Zyl, N. (2006). *Poverty and inequality in South Africa and the world*. Actuarial Society of South Africa.

Haughton, J., & Khandker, S. R. (2009). *Handbook on poverty and inequality*. World Bank.

Heslop, A., & Gorman, M. (2002). *Chronic poverty and older people in the developing world* (Working paper 10). Centre.

Kalomo, E. N., & Besthorn, F. H. (2018). Caregiving in Sub-Saharan Africa and older, female caregivers in the era of HIV/AIDS: A Namibian perspective. *Grand Families: The Contemporary Journal of Research, Practice and Policy, 5*(1), 33–48.

Kelly, G., Mrengqwa, L., & Geffen, L. (2019). "They don't care about us": Older people's experiences of primary healthcare in Cape Town, South Africa. *BMC Geriatrics, 19*(1), 1–14.

Kwan, C., & Walsh, C. A. (2018). Old age poverty: A scoping review of the literature. *Cogent Social Sciences, 4*(1), 1–21.

Leibbrandt, M., Poswell, L., Naidoo, P., & Welch, M. (2006). Measuring recent changes in South African inequality and poverty using 1996 and 2001

Census data. In H. Bhorat & R. Kanbur (Eds.), *Poverty and policy in post-apartheid South Africa*. Cape Town.

Lilenstein, K., Woolard, I., & Leibbrandt, M. (2016). *In-work poverty in South Africa: The impact of income sharing in the presence of high unemployment* (Southern Africa labour and development research unit working paper no 193). SALDRU, University of Cape Town.

Lin, I. F., Brown, S. L., & Hammersmith, A. M. (2017). Marital biography, social security receipt, and poverty. *Research on Aging, 39*(1), 86–110.

Lloyd-Sherlock, P., & Agrawal, S. (2014). Pensions and the health of older people in South Africa: Is there an effect? *The Journal of Development Studies, 50*(11), 1570–1586.

McLanahan, S. S., & Kelly, E. L. (2006). The feminization of poverty. In B. J. Risman & C. M. Froyum (Eds.), *Handbook of the sociology of gender*. Springer.

Moghadam, V. M. (2005). *The 'feminization of poverty' and women's human rights* (SHS papers in women's studies/gender research no 2). UNESCO.

Morris, A., & Hyslop, J. (1991). Education in South Africa: The present crisis and the problems of reconstruction. *Social Justice, 18*(43–44), 259–270.

Niño-Zarazúa, M., Barrientos, A., Hickey, S., & Hulme, D. (2012). Social protection in Sub-Saharan Africa: Getting the politics right. *World Development Journal, 40*(1), 163–176.

Nwosu, C. O., & Ndinda, C. (2018). Female household headship and poverty in South Africa: An employment-based analysis. *Economic Research Southern Africa, 3*(71), 1–26.

Patsios, D. (2006). *Pensioners, poverty and social exclusion: Poverty and social exclusion in Britain: The millennium survey*. Policy Press.

Pirrie, M., Harrison, L., Angeles, R., Marzanek, F., Ziesmann, A., & Agarwal, G. (2020). Poverty and food insecurity of older adults living in social housing in Ontario: A cross-sectional study. *BMC Public Health, 20*(1), 1–10.

Randel, J. (2017). *The ageing and development report: Poverty, independence and the world's older people*. HelpAge International.

Riumallo-Herl, C., Canning, D., & Kabudula, C. (2019). Health inequalities in the South African elderly: The importance of the measure of social-economic status. *The Journal of the Economics of Ageing, 14*, 1–16.

Rogan, M. (2018). Food poverty, hunger and household production in rural Eastern Cape households. *Development Southern Africa, 35*(1), 90–104.

SALDRU. (2019). *Overview wave 5 National Income Dynamics Survey (2008–2019)*. SALDRU.

Satumba, T., Bayat, A., & Mohamed, S. (2017). The impact of social grants on poverty reduction in South Africa. *Journal of Economics, 8*(1), 33–49.

Schatz, E., & Madhavan, S. (2011). Headship of older persons in the context of HIV/AIDS in rural South Africa. *African Population Studies, 25*(2), 1–16.

Sembene, D. (2015). *Poverty, growth, and inequality in Sub-Saharan Africa: Did the walk match the talk under the PRSP approach?* (International Monetary Fund working paper WP/15/122). IMF.

Smeeding, T. M., & Sandstrom, S. (2005). *Poverty and income maintenance in old age: A cross-national view of low income older women* (LIS working paper series no 398). Luxembourg Income Study (LIS).

South African Government. (2020). *Old age pension. About the older persons grant.* South African Government.

Statistics South Africa. (2008). *Measuring poverty in South Africa: Methodological report on the development of the poverty lines for statistical reporting.* Statistics South Africa.

Statistics South Africa. (2011). *Profile of older persons in South Africa.* Statistics South Africa.

Statistics South Africa. (2017a). *Poverty on the rise in South Africa.* Statistics South Africa.

Statistics South Africa. (2017b). *Poverty trends in South Africa - An examination of absolute poverty between 2006 and 2015.* Statistics South Africa.

Statistics South Africa. (2018a). *General household survey 2018. Statistical release P0310.* Statistics South Africa.

Statistics South Africa. (2018b). *National Poverty Lines. Statistical Release P0310.1.* Statistics South Africa.

Statistics South Africa. (2019). *National Poverty Lines 2019. Statistical release P0310.1.* Statistics South Africa.

Statistics South Africa. (2022). *Marginalised groups series VI: The social profile of older persons, 2017–2021.* Statistics South Africa.

Tanga, P., Tanga, M., & Gutura, P. (2019). The extended family support to older persons in the context of government social grant provisioning in South Africa. *Dirasat: Human and Social Sciences, 46*(1), 187–197.

Torres, S. (2014). Aging women, living poorer. *Contexts, 13*(2), 72–74.

UNDP. (2018). *Human development indices and indicators - 2018 statistical update.* Palgrave Macmillan.

UNDP. (2022). *South Africa National Human Development Report 2022: Harnessing the employability of South Africa's youth.* United Nations Development Program.

United Nations, Department of Economic and Social Affairs, Population Division (UNDESA). (2015a). *World population ageing 2015*. United Nations.

United Nations, Department of Economic and Social Affairs, Population Division (UNDESA). (2015b). *Income poverty in old age: An emerging development priority*. United Nations.

United Nations, Department of Economic and Social Affairs, Population Division (UNDESA). (2019a). *World population prospects: Highlights*. United Nations.

United Nations, Department of Economic and Social Affairs, Population Division (UNDESA). (2019b). *World population prospects: The 2019 revision*. United Nations.

Walker, C. (1990). *Women and gender in Southern Africa to 1945*. New Africa Books.

World Bank. (2015). *Global economic prospects. Regional outlook: Sub-Saharan Africa*. World Bank.

World Bank. (2018). *An incomplete transition: Overcoming the legacy of exclusion in South Africa*. World Bank.

World Health Organization (WHO). (2015). *World report on ageing and health*. World Health Organization.

5

Ageing in Anguish: Food Insecurity Dilemmas Confronting Older People

Themba Mgwaba and Pranitha Maharaj

Abstract Older people are often confronted by food insecurity dilemmas which compounds their health conditions. Drawing on 20 in-depth interviews with older adults from the Eastern Cape, South Africa, this study aimed at filling the gap in knowledge on food insecurity challenges confronting people aged 60 years and older. The interviews revealed that older people are confronted by various food availability, access, utilisation, and stability challenges. The peripheral nature of rural areas and limited shopping facilities largely explain food availability challenges facing most older adults. Since most poor older adults depend on government safety nets, often limited financial resources are the main cause of food access, utilisation, and stability dilemmas. A multifaceted strategy involving various players is needed to address the food insecurity dilemmas facing older people.

T. Mgwaba (✉) • P. Maharaj
School of Built Environment & Development Studies, University of KwaZulu-Natal, Durban, South Africa
e-mail: mgwabam@ukzn.ac.za; Maharajp7@ukzn.ac.za

P. Maharaj (ed.), *Navigating Ageing in South Africa*, Sustainable Development Goals Series, https://doi.org/10.1007/978-981-97-9088-3_5

Keywords Food insecurity; food access • Food availability • Older people • South Africa

Introduction

Food insecurity remains a major global concern, with more than 2 billion people worldwide suffering from moderate to severe food insecurity (FAO, 2023). Food insecurity is a term used to denote inadequate access to sufficient, safe, nutritious food to maintain an active and healthy life. Although hunger and food insecurity are closely related, hunger is defined as an unpleasant or painful physical experience brought on by inadequate food energy consumption (FAO, 2008). In 2020, 2.37 billion people worldwide lacked access to sufficient food, an increase of 320 million from the previous year (FAO, 2021). This was mostly because of lockdowns brought on by the global COVID-19 pandemic, which seriously disrupted food supply systems and resulted in a loss of revenue and livelihoods. The global pandemic also resulted in a global economic recession (Wade, 2023).

Increasingly, empirical evidence is suggesting a growing food insecurity challenge among older people around the world including South Africa (FAO, 2021; Statistics South Africa, 2019). One study found that in the United Kingdom an estimated 1.3 million adults aged 65 years and over are not eating enough protein while 34% of persons 65 years of age and older were found to be at risk of undernutrition upon hospital admission (Elia, 2015). According to more recent estimates from the Food and You Survey, 21% of adults in England experienced food insecurity in 2016 (Bates et al., 2017). Evidence indicates that undernutrition risk is increasing in the United Kingdom along with rising rates of food poverty, nevertheless, screening programmes for older adults have just recently been implemented (Bates et al., 2017; Elia, 2015). A study conducted in Canada found that, among aboriginal adults who live in food-insecure households, 36% were more likely to report poor general health versus 21% living in food-secure households (Willows et al., 2011).

The issue of food insecurity among the elderly is particularly serious in South Africa. At the national level, South Africa is food secure but at the household level food insecurity remains a major challenge (Oldewage-Theron & Egal, 2021). A national survey found that 14.2 million households out of almost 18 million households in 2021 had adequate access to food. However, 3.7 million indicated that they had inadequate access to food (Statistics South Africa, 2021). What is particularly challenging in the South African context is the limited information with respect to the extent of food insecurity challenges among older people (Denny et al., 2018). South Africa is food secure at a national level in that it produces enough food to meet its domestic needs. Nevertheless, high levels of poverty and inequality mean that there is a challenge around access to food, particularly nutritious food (Ziga & Karriem, 2022). In 2017, 21.3% of the South African households had either food inadequacy or severe food inadequacy challenges while 6.8 million South Africans were vulnerable to hunger (Statistics South Africa, 2019).

Food insecurity has become persistently high, driven mainly by the high prevalence of poverty in South Africa. Absolute poverty is incredibly high in South Africa. Although the country is classified as having a secure food supply, many households experience food insecurity and a high rate of undernutrition, primarily as a result of high rates of poverty and unemployment (Chakona & Shackleton, 2017). Food production is not the primary factor determining household food security in South Africa; rather, household income plays a significant role (Van den Berg & Walsh, 2023). Due to the belief that farming is a fall-back activity that should only be done when absolutely required and because others see the production of food as an indication of severe poverty, many South African households have given up on farming (Aliber & Hart, 2009). But by lowering reliance on purchased food, it has been demonstrated that home production increases the food security of low-income households in many places (Chakona & Shackleton, 2017).

Income, more than any other element, is critical to determining household food security in urban areas (Tawodzera, 2016). A decrease in household income or rise in food prices might have devastating effects leading to food insecurity in South Africa. According to Jacobs (2012), low-income households are more likely to experience food insecurity than middle-income and affluent households. A higher income allows households to make decisions about what to buy, how much to buy, where to buy it, and other food choices that lower-income households may not have access to (Tawodzera, 2016). Improving access to a steady and substantial source of income is thus an entry point for protection from food insecurity. Retirement, unemployment, or insufficient pension payments cause financial hardships for a large number of older South Africans. As a result, they struggle to provide a nutritious, wholesome, and well-balanced diet for themselves and dependents (Ogundeji, 2022), which is likely to have a negative impact on their health.

A study conducted in the United States of America found that there is a greater likelihood of chronic diseases (such as hypertension, heart disease, hepatitis, stroke, cancer, asthma, diabetes, arthritis, chronic obstructive pulmonary disease, and kidney disease) among adults in low food-secure households than high food-secure households (Gregory & Coleman-Jensen, 2017). When older individuals lack access to a sufficient supply of nutrient-rich food, their immune systems are compromised, they become more vulnerable to illness, and their general well-being is diminished. Among older people, food insecurity is linked to the onset or aggravation of chronic illnesses such diabetes, hypertension, and cardiovascular diseases. Elderly people's mental health might suffer from the stress and anxiety that comes with eating too little food, which can result in depression, social isolation, and a lower quality of life (Donini et al., 2003). Managing chronic conditions is likely to lead to increased financial burdens. These financial constraints frequently make it difficult for older persons who experience food insecurity to follow prescribed medical regimens (Fakoya et al., 2020).

Food insecurity among older people has become a major public policy challenge around the world due to the increasing number of older people and the precarious financial position in which they find themselves. Food insecurity, in general, remains an unabated global challenge and considering that older people are already a vulnerable group in society, it is reasonable to expect that they are most likely to be severely impacted. Food insecurity among older people is compounded by the distance involved in accessing food. Older people may reside in places where supermarkets or markets for fresh food are scarce or located some distance from their place of residence (Vilar-Compte et al., 2017). Grocery stores and markets that provide fresh and reasonably priced food are sometimes inaccessible to older people living in more remote areas. Their susceptibility to food instability is exacerbated by this lack of availability.

Older adults may find access to food particularly challenging due to ill health. Their financial resources are further strained by the expense of managing chronic disorders, which includes prescription drugs and specific diets, making it particularly challenging for them to get the nutrients they need. Food insecurity is more common among older people who live alone or do not have social support systems. It could be difficult for them to prepare meals, get access to food assistance programmes, or get support when they need it (Oldewage-Theron & Egal, 2021). A further factor contributing to food insecurity among older adults is the lack of availability of nutrient-dense food options, particularly in rural or low-income locations (Bowen et al., 2022). Because of age-related health issues, older adults frequently have particular nutritional needs. Their medical issues may necessitate that they adhere to specific diets, which can be costly and difficult to follow, making food insecurity worse.

People can experience food insecurity to varying degrees, depending on a variety of demographic characteristics, including whether or not they are hungry. Insufficient food can lead to hunger, a distressing feeling that impacts a large number of the elderly, particularly those from a poorer background. Hunger is a grave concern because of the age-related decline in health and the prevalence of chronic diseases. For non-communicable diseases like type 2 diabetes and hypertension, the consequences of poor health are more severe for older persons. Due to its effect on mental health in general, food insecurity has also been connected to negative mental health outcomes (Jones, 2017).

When compared to older adults who have access to food, those who experience food insecurity report reduced nutritious intake, worse health, higher levels of sadness, and difficulty carrying out daily life activities (De Andrade et al., 2009). In terms of oral health, chewing ability and eating can be impacted by dental issues discomfort, and the usage of dental prostheses. This may restrict the options for nutritious meals, increasing the risk of malnutrition and contributing to a lower standard of living (De Andrade et al., 2009). Food insecurity among older adults and the associated adverse health outcomes tend to be more severe and often intensify the necessity for health care services (Bhargava & Lee, 2016;

Samodien et al., 2021). Older people who are already weak are more prone to illnesses if they experience food insecurity. As a result, their morbidity and death rates increase due to the body's increased requirement for nutrition during illness (Shetty, 2009).

With over 21% of the population suffering from acute food insecurity, Sub-Saharan Africa continues to be one of the most afflicted regions (Militao et al., 2022; Simelane & Oosthuizen, 2023). Food insecurity is very common in Southern Africa because of a number of issues including poverty, climate change, and economic hardship. Recent research show that about 8% of the population is elderly in South Africa (Statistics South Africa, 2023). Older people in South Africa are thought to be particularly vulnerable to food insecurity (Bain et al., 2013), yet very little is known about their experience of food security (Denny et al., 2018). The COVID-19 pandemic has weakened efforts to achieve the National Development Plans and the UN Sustainable Development Goals (SDGs) of zero hunger by 2030, as well as depriving many South Africans of their constitutionally guaranteed right to sufficient food.

The food insecurity challenges facing adults must be understood in a two-pronged manner. Firstly, the number of older people in the population in South Africa is rapidly growing. According to Statistics South Africa (2023), there were about five million people age 60 and above in 2022. Secondly, older people struggle financially as a result of retirement, fewer job prospects, and absence of pension plans. Food insecurity results from their inability to afford a healthy diet due to their limited or low income (Vilar-Compte et al., 2017). The mere fact that more elderly people are living on fixed incomes from social security or pensions, which may not be enough to cover all of their expenses, including food, is one of the primary causes of the rise in food insecurity. There is no doubt that food insecurity is a serious problem that affects people everywhere, especially the elderly. Considering that most food insecurity studies are largely quantitative in nature and tend to omit older people, the aim of this chapter is to use qualitative research methods to unravel the food insecurity challenges and/or dilemmas confronting older people.

Food Security in the Eastern Cape

Using a qualitative inquiry, this chapter focuses on food insecurity experiences among older people in the Eastern Cape. It explores how older people are affected by food insecurity challenges using four hierarchical dimensions of food insecurity: availability, access, utilisation, and stability. Food insecurity is higher in the Eastern Cape than other provinces (Cheteni et al., 2020). The vast majority of the population in the province reside in rural areas, especially older people. Almost 72% of the population resides in rural areas, with a staggering 70% of these individuals facing poverty (Ngumbela et al., 2020). The Eastern Cape is the poorest and fourth most populous province in South Africa (Statistics South Africa, 2023). The province suffers from structural poverty which emanates from the ugly apartheid history of Bantustans which meant that less resources were allocated for the development of these provinces (Ngumbela et al., 2020).

Most households in the province fall in the food poverty line with the majority of these households relying on government social grants to make ends meet (Cheteni et al., 2020). The Eastern Cape is the most food insecure province, with four out of every five households experiencing hunger, making women and children especially vulnerable to its impacts (Maraisa et al., 2022). The automobile manufacturing industry is the backbone of the economy of the Eastern Cape; however, the majority of the population earn their livelihood in the informal sector (Ngumbela et al., 2020). The province is heavily impacted by changing weather patterns, resulting in severe hardships for many households and families, especially those residing in rural areas (Amoah, 2021). These difficulties often manifest as extreme poverty, scarcity of water, and uncertainty regarding food availability. This study is conducted against the backdrop of abject poverty which confronts the majority of the population in Eastern Cape and the empirical evidence suggesting that most previous food security studies have tended to focus on predominantly urban provinces, at the exclusion of rural provinces such as Eastern Cape (Cheteni et al., 2020). Drawing from 20 in-depth interviews with older people, this study aimed at filling the gap in knowledge on food insecurity challenges facing older people in Eastern Cape, South Africa.

All 20 study participants were over 60 years old, with an equal proportion of men and women. The majority of the study participants (12) were in the 60–69 age group, with the remaining participants (8) aged 70 and over. Most (15) of the study participants were married. All were dependent on the old age social grant as their main source of income. Most (18) study participants had primary or secondary education. Only two had completed their secondary school education. Data was analysed using the thematic analysis approach by repeatedly reading the interview transcripts; identifying and coding emerging themes; and merging similar themes. Most studies conducted on food insecurity matters have been predominantly quantitative in nature using different types of scales to measure it: food insecurity experience scale (FIES); household food insecurity access scale (HFIAS); household hunger scale (HHS); and others. This has led to a general neglect of the voices of the affected people, especially the most vulnerable groups such as older people. It is therefore the intention of the study to illuminate the food insecurity discourse through thick verbal descriptions provided by older people. To this end, an effort has been made to bring forth the voice of the participants using verbatim quotations from of the research participants. By capturing the voices of participants this study succeeds in giving an *emic* (inside-out) perspective of day-to-day food insecurity struggles confronting older people in the Eastern Cape.

Food Availability

There is a multiplicity of food insecurity challenges facing older people and according to Sengupta (2016) include a decline in food consumption, reduction in food supply, and limited access. Food availability refers to a reliable and consistent source of sufficient quality food for an active and healthy life (Ashby et al., 2016). Food availability is realised when people have enough food of sufficient nutritional quality (Gross et al., 2000). Food availability is therefore understood, in the main, as referring to the extent of food production at different levels, that is, global, national, community, household, and individual levels. The availability of food may depend on home subsistence farming initiatives, as well as transport systems to ensure food is conveniently available to the population at large (Ashby et al., 2016).

Food availability amongst older people living in peripheral areas in Eastern Cape is limited largely because food is usually sourced from informal traders, also known as spaza shops. There are three main reasons to explain why older people buy their food from these informal traders instead of large supermarkets in town. Firstly, the transport costs to get to town, where large food supermarkets are available, is a major deterrent for older people who do not have the funds to pay for taxi fares. Secondly, local spaza shop owners extend credit facilities to the elderly especially as they are likely to run out of food closer to grant paydays. In this way older people live in a debt-trap which is crucial for their own survival on the one hand and designed to ensure the survival of spaza shops on the other hand. The challenge however is that spaza shops do not always have all the food items which older people would like to purchase. These shops only offer a limited range of food products, which means that the elderly are not able to meet their dietary requirements. They have to make do with what is available in the community. One elderly woman explains: *"We get food from local spaza shops (informal traders) and pay later when we have money, we do not get everything from these shops and some of the items you want will not be available and you will buy something else you did not mean to buy"*. The poor quality of food often sold by spaza shop owners are a cause for concern. Thirdly, most spaza shops have invented a mechanism to deliver food at the doorstep of these poor households thereby solving transport challenges facing older people. These efforts by spaza shops could be lauded on the one hand since they help solve transport and logistical challenges facing older people in accessing food. However, on the other hand, these efforts should be seen for what they are, that is, as another trap to ensure that destitute older people continue accessing food from spaza shops which stock limited food items with questionable quality standards which allow spaza shop owners to sustain their businesses through guaranteed and stable turnover derived from older people. The comment from one older woman echoed these sentiments: *"I get my food from spaza shops and sometimes in town when I am in town. I do not face any challenges when it comes to costs of transportation because the owners of these spaza shops they bring them to your house, and you do not have to be worried about transportation".* The quality of food from spaza shops is often compromised in the sense that they sell foods that extend beyond their shelf life and sold by these informal traders to the community. The consequential health hazards emanating from consuming expired food items cannot be exaggerated especially considering that it is older people who are consuming such foods. An older woman explained this: *"so they do not have all food items like fresh meat, and someone advised me to go to town because most of the times these spaza shops are selling expired food, yet I do not always have money to go to town".*

In rural, and remote areas, personal and environmental factors may lead to unequal access in health resources and can either promote or hinder healthy eating (Casey et al., 2008). Vulnerable populations, such as older adults, may find it difficult to get the food necessary for a healthy diet. The limited range of food items available from the spaza shops may therefore aggravate the health conditions of the elderly. In one of the interviews, a participant revealed the essence of what older people, with special dietary requirements, have to go through: *"Yes, I have special dietary requirements, I do not eat food that contains too much sugar like cakes and other sweet things like chocolate. I eat a lot because I am using a treatment that influences my appetite. However, I do not get the food that I need to manage my diabetes".* Food insecurity dilemmas may therefore exacerbate the management of chronic diseases in the sense that poorer older people often cannot afford a special diet.

Food Access

Food access is related to the need for the resources required in order to put food on the table which could be economic or physical. It refers to the food needed by all household members to meet their dietary requirements and food preferences and to achieve and maintain optimal nutritional status (Ashby et al., 2016). Access to food in the main relates to the financial ability to afford appropriate foods for a nutritious diet (FAO, 2006). Older people are experiencing a great deal of financial difficulties which in turn directly impacts negatively on their access to food. Most older people often live with dependents, usually grandchildren and sometimes extended family members. These dependents often live off the limited old age social grant that is meant to take care of older people. In the Eastern Cape, like much of the country, unemployment is very high. One elderly woman stated: *"Yes, I share food with my sister's children, they usually come to me when they need something to eat, and I give them. However, this makes me run out of food earlier and I find myself without food"*.

A growing percentage of older people are facing financial constraints as a result of their poverty status, with many of them missing meals. Older adults might hide their situation from others. Many try to ensure their children and grandchildren eat enough food, while they themselves go hungry (Purdam et al., 2019). Most older people are unemployed, and the old age grant is their only source of income. However, the very limited income they have has to be spent on other important needs such as medical services and funeral covers. Older people seek healthcare often because of their deteriorating health. The free healthcare available in public health facilities (clinics and hospitals) is besieged with many challenges and the main one is overcrowding and poor quality of services. Consequently, public health facilities are avoided up until one cannot avoid them when they are seriously ill. Older people, understandably so, spend their limited financial resources planning for their funeral expenses. The following statement from an older man explains it: *"The amount of money that I receive is very small to meet my needs, the food I buy is not enough because I have to pay funeral cover, which is R250 per month, and I also have debts that I make during the month when I want to buy some food items. If I was in good health, I was going to do small jobs, but I cannot because I am suffering from asthma"*. Hence some older people, if they were given a chance, would rather work to get extra income but they are not able to do so because their health conditions do not permit them.

Food is considered expensive by most older people since they are depending on their old age grants to buy food to last them for the entire month. Most run out of food before month end or before their next grant payday. They cannot afford to buy the healthy food they need, and they cannot rely on support, in the form of remittances, from family members of working-age due to the high unemployment rates in South Africa. This statement from an elderly woman attest to this phenomenon: *"Yes, the food that I am supposed to eat should not have too much oil, salt, and spice because those things are not right for my health. I am unable to get the food that is good for my health because no one is supporting me".*

There is a limited access to food among older people in Eastern Cape. Older people living in peripheral areas face serious challenges accessing food because of transport costs. One elderly man explained: *"I buy food in town and check which shop have better prices because I do not have a specific shop, I buy anywhere in town. There are challenges that I face, for example, transport that needs to be paid and sometimes I do not have money at that moment because I get my money in town. But how do I get to town in order to get my money?"* Since destitute older people rely on government old age social grants as their only or main source of income, even transport costs that may seem reasonable to the general public may prove difficult to afford for them. In this way, transport costs serve as one of the barriers to accessing food for older people. Over and above transport costs, the scarcity of transport alternatives prevalent in remote rural areas often exacerbate food access dilemmas confronting older people residing in these areas. One older woman explained: *"I use public transport, we have a car in our village that works from 5am to 10pm every day, and we depend on it. I buy food in town and in spaza shops that are near me. There are challenges that I am facing like transport because if you miss a car at 5am it will be difficult to get transport and you will have to wait till the next day".*

Food Utilisation

Food utilisation refers to the consumption of sufficient and safe food which meets the nutritional and physiological needs of the individuals (Barrett, 2010). It also refers to physical, social, and human resources required to transform food into proper meals and encompasses food safety achieved by sanitary and hygienic conditions (Abosede, 2020). Food utilisation depends on people's ability to source nutritionally adequate foods and their ability and resources to safely prepare and store them (Barrett, 2010). Older people, owing to their physical frailty, are confronted with human resources challenges which renders it difficult to transform food into meals. Age and chronic illnesses are associated with a higher chance of having a functional limitation, which may impact a person's ability to leave the house and get assistance with eating (Dunlop et al., 2002). Often older people are short of people to assist them with food preparation, and as a result, they either have to do this themselves even at advanced age or risk going hungry even when food is available at the house. One elderly woman noted: *"I have my children here, but they are not always with me because they are still looking for jobs. Sometimes I do not have someone to prepare food for me. However, I do what I can do, for example, I cook and eat what I have, and it could be anything that is available".*

The other challenge confronting destitute older people is lack of required food storage facilities such as refrigerators. In resource constrained settings, such as rural areas, owning a fridge is a luxury; hence, most older people residing in these settings do not own refrigerators which in turn threatens food availability and promotes food wastage. In some instances, their refrigerator is not functioning and they do not have the funds to either repair it or purchase a new one. For example, this statement from an elderly man explains it: *"I use buckets to store food but there are other types of food that needs to be in the fridge and I store them in the fridge. I dispose of food when they are bad especially when my fridge is not working, for example my fridge is currently not working and there are food items that will be rotten and I have no choice but to dispose of them.* The challenge of intermittent power cuts, known as load-shedding, has severe negative consequences on food storage in South Africa. As a result of load-shedding, appliances such as refrigerators may malfunction, resulting in food that needs to be kept in cool temperatures being spoiled. The following statement from an elderly man in Eastern Cape highlights the plight of the poor in the face of intermittent power cuts in South Africa: *"I store my food well because I have a fridge so that when I buy things like vegetables, I keep it in the fridge, and I also have other ways of keeping other food items like mealie meal on shelves until the month ends. However, the vegetables do not sustain us for the whole month, but I have a way of keeping other items fresh. Due to load-shedding or disruption of electricity for a long time we have to dispose of food because at that time the food is bad. So yes, I dispose of food".* Inadequate electricity supply is negatively impacting older people with limited resources by forcing them to dispose of food because it is spoiled. This is severely impacting their ability to meet their nutritional and physiological needs.

Food Stability

Food stability denotes appreciation that access to food is transitory, cyclical, or chronic. Food stability over time affects the three aforementioned dimensions of food security through seasonal and temporary change (Gross et al., 2000). Food insecurity therefore may occur when availability, access to, and utilisation of safe, culturally appropriate and nutritious food is compromised, or when these foods cannot be obtained through socially acceptable means. Food stability is threatened and compromised owing to adverse weather conditions, climate change, rising food prices, political or civil conflicts, or other catastrophes including economic factors like unemployment (Carletto et al., 2013; Ecker & Breisinger, 2012).

The world has recently experienced the global COVID-19 pandemic and South Africa was not spared in its disastrous effects especially on food price hikes. The pandemic disrupted food supply systems and resulted in a global economic downturn (World Bank, 2024). Moreover, natural disasters such as droughts and floods have been more pronounced in South Africa in the recent past than any other years. All these factors combined have had a direct effect on food supply, by reducing or disrupting it, and thereby leading to upward pressure on food prices.

The prices of food items have also soared while social grants have been increasing at below inflation rate in the last few years. The increase of social grants in a diminishing rate, and below inflation rate, means older people have less purchasing power to meet their needs. Older people find food items more expensive than ever before and as a result have to make some adjustments in terms of their dietary requirements. The latter is succinctly captured in the following statement by an elderly woman: *"There are food items that I want but I do not afford them like vegetables, I do not even afford to buy cosmetics which are also expensive, so the little money I have will buy food that is not even good quality. This really affects me because I cannot eat what I want because the amount of money I have is used for attending other household problems. Yes, there are food items I would like to buy like cabbage, potatoes and other vegetables".*

In the quest to live within their means, older people have had to revise their spending patterns and as a result, they sacrifice healthy foods (e.g. fruits and vegetables) and opt to buy less nutritious foods instead, to avoid going hungry. Moreover, older people resort to buying food that is of a lower quality so that they have the required quantity to last until the next payday. Poor quality foods may negatively affect the already compromised older people's health status (Ngumbela et al., 2020). Lower income households consume fewer fruits and vegetables than higher income households (Battersby & Watson, 2019; Blekking et al., 2020). Nutritious foods, particularly vegetables and fruits, are a necessity for the wellbeing of the people, particularly older people, yet these food items are not a priority due to financial constraints (Cheteni et al., 2020; Selepe et al., 2015).

Some of the Coping Strategies

In an effort to mitigate the devastating impact of food insecurity, older people resort to culturally and socially embedded practices such as sharing of food when it runs out. These practices resonate with the Afrocentric philosophy of *ubuntu* which has been well propounded by various scholars and cultural experts. *Ubuntu* in essence literally means humanity; however, at a deeper philosophical level it means 'a person is a person through other people' which suggests that people cannot exist and prosper in isolation from others. It is this philosophy which propagates communal distribution of wealth rather than individualistic centred prosperity. The practice of food sharing should, however, be seen for what it is. Although it is a coping survival strategy, it is actually the poor helping the poor and this happens because of the vacuum created by the absence of effective government or civil society driven safety nets on such important areas as food insecurity. The following statement from an elderly woman captures the dilemma and inherent contradictions in implementing these coping strategies: *"I eat three times per day. Yes, there are those times when I will spend a day without eating anything because I have no food to eat. Sometimes, I ask other people to share small food items so that when I have food, I can pay them back, and they help, and sometimes they do not*". Lending of food, however, proves to be an unreliable coping strategy because often the people they rely on for assistance are also poor and as such are not always in a position to help. Consequently, older people find themselves having to go without food, in some, if not most, instances.

In an effort to alleviate hunger and poverty, older people engage in stokvels—an informal savings pool in which funds are contributed in rotation, allowing participants access to lump sums for family needs, including funeral expenses or other important events. Stokvels are an informal saving collective initiative mainly found in developing countries due to their large-scale exclusion from the formal financial sector. These collectives fall under the framework of the Rotating Savings and Credit Associations (ROSCAs) (Lappeman et al., 2020). Some recent research indicates that there are 11.4 million South Africans belonging to 811,130 stokvels, which have a collective value of R49 billion a year (Lappeman et al., 2020; Mfeti, 2017). Stokvels are used for a variety of purposes, for example, credit, food, as well as burial cover (Lappeman et al., 2020). Research also shows that stokvels play a vital role in food security matters especially in rural areas through amassing purchasing power and facilitating access to bulk discounts (Lappeman et al., 2020; Lukwa et al., 2024). All these initiatives put a strain on the already exhausted social grant and render disposable income smaller. The following statement from an elderly man echoes these sentiments: "*There are things like (umgalelo) financial supports we do to help each other for extra money. The people I live with here need to be fed, but this affects my ability to get enough food at the same time. We have stokvels in our community, so you are expected to contribute to the stokvel. We pay R500 per month, and all those efforts are just for funeral services*".

Conclusion

In conclusion, food insecurity among the elderly is a multifaceted dilemma with wide-ranging effects. A multifaceted strategy involving social welfare programmes, community-based initiatives, governmental reforms, and education is needed to address the challenge of food insecurity among older people. The general well-being and quality of life of the elderly can be raised by putting their needs first and making sure they have access to enough nourishing food. Governments, organisations, and communities must collaborate to fight food insecurity among the elderly. Food insecurity is a complicated challenge that has serious negative effects on the health and wellbeing of older adults in South Africa. In order to reduce food insecurity and enhance the quality of life of older people in South Africa, certain solutions can be put into place, such as community-based initiatives, social welfare programmes, and education campaigns. In order to support older people's general health and dignity, it is imperative that stakeholders at all levels collaborate to guarantee that they have access to inexpensive, nutrient-rich food.

Interventions in the public health sector is much needed. Frontline staff such as doctors, physician assistants, nurses, clinical pharmacists, and health specialists should be sensitive to ailments emanating from food insecurity and malnutrition and conduct a thorough patient examination in this regard. Referrals to appropriate government departments such as the Department of Social Development and Department of Agriculture should be made in the event of malnutrition and/or food insecurity being detected as the root cause of ailments. It is important that an effective inter-governmental plan between the various sectors is designed and implemented with speed.

Health centres and providers should rely on intervention tools that properly assess their capacity to implement transformative initiatives among their patients while considering their social determinants of health, given the projected growth of older adults and the rising demand for interventions to meet the needs of this population (Vincent et al., 2014). This is crucial in order to properly recommend clients to social workers and better support senior citizens in locating a food bank in their community. Some strategies that can help in reducing food insecurity among older people are the social welfare programmes which are financial aid initiatives that governments might put in place to help elderly citizens buy wholesome food. Non-governmental organisations and community groups can also create food assistance programmes, like food banks, meal delivery services, and community gardens, with an emphasis on the elderly. The establishment of age-friendly dietary regulations, greater financing for social assistance programmes, and better access to healthcare services are a few examples of policy reforms that advocacy groups should concentrate on in order to better meet the requirements of senior citizens.

Other social assistance programmes may include social safety nets like food vouchers or cash transfers which will afford older people access to wholesome food and financial support. Encouraging sustainable farming could also help and older farmers stand to gain from the promotion of sustainable farming methods including conservation agriculture and agroforestry, which can increase agricultural productivity and climate change resilience. As older people are vulnerable to diseases, improving access to health care services, providing dietary advice, and routine check-ups can assist in addressing health issues linked to food insecurity. Education campaigns and creating awareness is critical to increase public knowledge of the problem of food insecurity among the elderly.

The government of South Africa has the authority to establish or improve social welfare programmes that are specifically designed to aid the elderly population. These programmes offer financial support to meet their basic needs, which includes access to wholesome meals. It is imperative to design comprehensive plans to alleviate food insecurity among older people, through cooperation between governmental and non-governmental organisations as well as endeavouring to put practical solutions into practice.

References

Abosede, S. (2020). Water, food security, and trade in Sub-Saharan Africa. In V. Erokhin & T. Gao (Eds.), *Handbook of research on globalized agricultural trade and new challenges for food security*. Pennsylvania.

Aliber, M., & Hart, T. G. (2009). Should subsistence agriculture be supported as a strategy to address rural food insecurity? *Agrekon, 48*(4), 434–458.

Amoah, L. N. A. (2021). Water scarcity and food security in Ngqeleni locality in the Eastern Cape Province-South Africa. *African Journal of Hospitality, Tourism and Leisure, 10*, 40–53.

Ashby, S., Kleve, S., McKechnie, R., & Palermo, C. (2016). Measurement of the dimensions of food insecurity in developed countries: A systematic literature review. *Public Health Nutrition, 19*(16), 2887–2896.

Bain, L. E., Awah, P. K., Geraldine, N., Kindong, N. P., Siga, Y., Bernard, N., & Tanjeko, A. T. (2013). Malnutrition in sub—Saharan Africa: Burden, causes and prospects. *The Pan African Medical Journal, 15*(1), 120.

Barrett, C. B. (2010). Measuring food insecurity. *Science, 327*, 825–828.

Bates, B., Roberts, C., Lepps, H., & Porter, L. (2017). *The food and you survey wave 4*. Food Standards Agency.

Battersby, J., & Watson, V. (2019). *Urban food systems governance and poverty in African cities*. Taylor & Francis.

Bhargava, V., & Lee, J. S. (2016). Food insecurity and health care utilization among older adults in the United States. *Journal of Nutrition in Gerontology and Geriatrics, 35*(3), 177–192.

Blekking, J., Waldman, K., Tuholske, C., & Evans, T. (2020). Formal/informal employment and urban food security in Sub-Saharan Africa. *Applied Geography, 114*, 102131.

Bowen, S., Elliott, S., & Hardison-Moody, A. (2022). Rural food insecurity: A longitudinal analysis of low-income rural households with children in the south. RSF: The Russell Sage Foundation. *Journal of the Social Sciences, 8*(3), 50–77.

Carletto, C., Zezza, A., & Banerjee, R. (2013). Towards better measurement of household food security: Harmonizing indicators and the role of household surveys. *Global Food Security, 2*, 30–40.

Casey, A. A., Elliott, M., Glanz, K., Haire-Joshu, D., Lovegreen, S. L., Saelens, B. E., Sallis, J. F., & Brownson, R. C. (2008). Impact of the food and physical activity environments on behaviours and weight status in rural U.S. communities. *Preventive Medicine, 47*, 600–604.

Chakona, G., & Shackleton, C. M. (2017). Local setting influences the quantity of household food waste in mid-sized South African towns. *PLoS One, 12*(12), e0189407.

Cheteni, P., Khamfula, Y., & Mah, G. (2020). Exploring food security and household dietary diversity in the Eastern Cape Province, South Africa. *Sustainability, 12*(5), 1851.

De Andrade, F. B., De França Caldas, A., & Kitoko, P. M. (2009). Relationship between oral health, nutrient intake and nutritional status in a sample of Brazilian elderly people. *Gerodontology, 26*(1), 40–45.

Denny, R. C., Marquart-Pyatt, S. T., Ligmann-Zielinska, A., Olabisi, L. S., Rivers, L., Du, J., & Liverpool-Tasie, L. S. O. (2018). Food security in Africa: A cross-scale, empirical investigation using structural equation modelling. *Environment Systems and Decisions, 38*, 6–22.

Donini, L., Savina, C., & Cannella, C. (2003). Eating habits and appetite control in the elderly: The anorexia of aging. *International Psychogeriatrics, 15*(1), 73–87.

Dunlop, D. D., Manheim, L. M., Sohn, M. W., Liu, X., & Chang, R. W. (2002). Incidence of functional limitation in older adults: The impact of gender, race, and chronic conditions. *Archives of Physical Medicine and Rehabilitation, 83*(7), 964–971.

Ecker, O., & Breisinger, C. (2012). *The food security system: A new conceptual framework*. International Food Policy Research Institute.

Elia, M. (2015). *The cost of malnutrition in England and potential cost Savings from nutritional interventions* (Annual report). British Association of Parenteral and Enteral Nutrition.

Fakoya, O. A., McCorry, N. K., & Donnelly, M. (2020). Loneliness and social isolation interventions for older adults: A scoping review of reviews. *BMC Public Health, 20*, 1–14.

Food and Agriculture Organization (FAO). (2006). *The state of food security and nutrition in the world*. Food & Agriculture Organization.

Food and Agriculture Organization (FAO). (2008). *The state of food security and nutrition in the world*. Food & Agriculture Organization.

Food and Agriculture Organization (FAO). (2021). *The state of food security and nutrition in the world*. Food & Agriculture Organization.

Food and Agriculture Organization (FAO). (2023). *The state of food security and nutrition in the world (SOFI)*. Food & Agriculture Organization.

Gregory, C. A., & Coleman-Jensen, A. (2017). *Food insecurity, chronic disease, and Health among working-age adults* (Rural status report). Hansa Digital and Litho Printers.

Gross, R., Schoeneberger, H., Pfeifer, H., & Preuss, H. J. (2000). *Four dimensions of food and nutrition security: Definitions and concepts*. UN/AAC Subcommittee on Nutrition.

Jacobs, P. (2012). Household food insecurity, rapid food price inflation and the economic downturn in South Africa. *Agenda, 24*(86), 38–51.

Jones, A. D. (2017). Food insecurity and mental health status: A global analysis of 149 countries. *American Journal of Preventive Medicine, 53*(2), 264–273.

Lappeman, J., Litkie, J., Bramdaw, S., & Quibell, A. (2020). Exploring retail orientated rotating savings and credit associations: Festive season 'stokvels' in South Africa. *The International Review of Retail, Distribution and Consumer Research, 30*(3), 331–358.

Lukwa, A. T., Wayas, F. A., Lambert, E. V., "Savings for Health" IDRC Collaborators, & Alaba, O. (2024). Stakeholder mapping to explore social and economic capital of Rotating Savings and Credit Associations (ROSCAs) to increase demand for and access to healthy food. *Frontiers in Sustainable Food Systems, 8*.

Maraisa, M. L., Lessing, E., & Frank, T. (2022). Assessment of the realisation of the right to adequate food in the Blue Crane Route (Eastern Cape, South Africa). *South African Journal of Clinical Nutrition, 35*(3), 122–132.

Mfeti, T. (2017). *Stokvels: The power of a collective*. https://www.sanlam.co.za/mediacentre/media-category/media-releases/Stokvels%20-%20The%20Power%20of%20a%20Collective

Militao, E. M., Salvador, E. M., Uthman, O. A., Vinberg, S., & Macassa, G. (2022). Food insecurity and health outcomes other than malnutrition in Southern Africa: A descriptive systematic review. *International Journal of Environmental Research and Public Health, 19*(9), 5082.

Ngumbela, X. G., Khalema, E. N., & Nzimakwe, T. I. (2020). Local worlds: Vulnerability and food insecurity in the Eastern Cape province of South Africa. *Jàmbá: Journal of Disaster Risk Studies, 12*(1), 1–10.

Ogundeji, A. A. (2022). Adaptation to climate change and impact on smallholder farmers' food security in South Africa. *Agriculture, 12*(5), 589.

Oldewage-Theron, W., & Egal, A. A. (2021). Is food insecurity a problem among the elderly in Sharpeville, South Africa? *Food Security, 13*(1), 71–81.

Purdam, K., Esmail, A., & Garratt, E. (2019). Food insecurity amongst older people in the UK. *British Food Journal, 121*(3), 658–674.

Samodien, E., Abrahams, Y., Muller, C., Louw, J., & Chellan, N. (2021). Non-communicable diseases-a catastrophe for South Africa. *South African Journal of Science, 117*(5–6), 1–6.

Selepe, B. M., Mtyingizane, S. S., & Masuku, M. M. (2015). Factors contributing to household food insecurity in Mhlontlo area, Eastern Cape, South Africa. *African Journal of Hospitality, Tourism and Leisure, 4*(1), 1–11.

Sengupta, P. (2016). Food security among the elderly: An area of concern. *Journal of Gerontology and Geriatric Research, 5*, 9–10.

Shetty, P. (2009). Incorporating nutritional considerations when addressing food insecurity. *Food Security, 1*(4), 431–440.

Simelane, T., & Oosthuizen, A. (2023). HSRC survey indicates need for area-specific interventions for food and nutrition security in South Africa. *Human Sciences Research Council Review, 21*(4), 38–41.

Statistics South Africa. (2019). *Towards measuring food security in South Africa: An examination of hunger and food inadequacy*. Statistics South Africa.

Statistics South Africa. (2021). *General household survey*. Statistics South Africa.

Statistics South Africa. (2023). *Census 2022*. Statistics South Africa.

Tawodzera, G. (2016). Food insecurity in a state in crisis. In J. Crush & J. Battersby (Eds.), *Rapid urbanisation, urban food deserts and food security in Africa*. Springer.

Van den Berg, L., & Walsh, C. M. (2023). Household food insecurity in South Africa from 1999 to 2021: A metrics perspective. *Public Health Nutrition, 26*, 1–17.

Vilar-Compte, M., Gaitán-Rossi, P., & Pérez-Escamilla, R. (2017). Food insecurity measurement among older adults: Implications for policy and food security governance. *Global Food Security, 14*, 87–95.

Vincent, H. K., Vincent, K. R., Seay, A. N., Conrad, B. P., Hurley, R. W., & George, S. Z. (2014). Back strength predicts walking improvement in obese, older adults with chronic low back pain. *PM&R, 6*(5), 418–426.

Wade, R. H. (2023). The world development report 2022: Finance for an equitable recovery in the context of the international debt crisis. *Development and Change, 54*(5), 1354–1373.

Willows, N., Veugelers, P., Raine, K., & Kuhle, S. (2011). Associations between household food insecurity and health outcomes in the Aboriginal population (excluding reserves). *Health Reports, 22*(2), 15.

World Bank. (2024). *Food security update*. World Bank.

Ziga, M., & Karriem, A. (2022). NCD prevention through an equitable food system in South Africa: Opportunities and challenges. *ESR Review: Economic and Social Rights in South Africa, 23*(4), 7–12.

6

Reciprocity of Support in the Family: Perspective of Older Persons

Siyamthanda Jordaan and Pranitha Maharaj

Abstract As people grow older, there is a greater need for care and support. Families often play an important role in the provision of support, shelter, and care for older people in South Africa. The focus of this chapter is to understand the lived experiences of older people in providing and receiving care in South Africa. The study draws on interviews with 20 older people living in a township in South Africa. Children play an important role in taking care of the health care needs of their parents, especially if they are in a position to provide financial support. However, older adults do not want to burden their children, unless absolutely necessary. They would rather draw on their own resources before turning to their children for support. Older people are not a burden but sometimes a valuable source of care provision. Some feel that they are left with no choice because they are the only ones with the means to provide support within their homes and sometimes communities. Older people are

S. Jordaan (✉) • P. Maharaj
School of Built Environment and Development Studies, University of KwaZulu-Natal, Durban, South Africa
e-mail: Maharajp7@ukzn.ac.za

P. Maharaj (ed.), *Navigating Ageing in South Africa*, Sustainable Development Goals Series, https://doi.org/10.1007/978-981-97-9088-3_6

dependent on family members for support, but they also provide support to others, particularly for young members of their households.

Keywords Family • Care • Support • Reciprocity • South Africa

Introduction

Elderly care in South Africa is a growing concern due to the country's rapidly ageing population. In the absence of affordable formal care systems outside of the health sector, the responsibility for elder care often falls on family members (WHO, 2015a, b, c). Families have long served as the main provider of support, shelter, and care for the elderly in South Africa. As individuals age, family relationships often become much more critical; in addition, their need for care increases, and other social connections including in the workplace become less prominent in their lives (Thomas et al., 2017). Families frequently have common values, beliefs, and traditions, which fosters a sense of unity and belonging (Bengtson & Martin, 2001). Moreover, a deep emotional connection is a key factor that keeps families together (Świderska, 2014). Families often share experiences, both joyful and sad, which fosters shared memories and strengthens bonds (Świderska, 2014). As people age, they have a stronger need for security and belonging than in earlier years of life. With ageing come changes in the type of reciprocal exchange of benefits and services between generations. Research suggests that people who are aged 65–69 years tend to provide more for their adult children than the children do for them. However, around the age of 75, people become more dependent on their children for support (WHO, 2015a, b, c), especially with activities of daily living. Older adults and their children who live together or close by, often exchange benefits and resources on a significantly larger and more frequent basis (Wang et al., 2020).

Ageing is associated with an increased need for care, assistance, and health services. As people live longer, they are more likely to experience chronic conditions such as diabetes, cardiovascular diseases, and stroke-related impairments. Physical, psychological, and social health issues are frequently associated with ageing and have become more complex and interconnected (WHO, 2002). As people age, they may also require more assistance with their daily activities and they are also less able to contribute physically to their household (Kengne & Mayosi, 2014). Moreover, they are less likely to perform strenuous activities such as farming, collecting water or firewood, and taking care of themselves or others within their households (Kengne & Mayosi, 2014). Their ability to perform fundamental tasks necessary for daily living is frequently hampered by functional decline and physical reliance that come with ageing. In this context, the family has an important role to play in the support and care given to older people.

Poverty, circular migration, and the impact of HIV/AIDS all contribute to poor elderly care in South Africa (Lehohla, 2014). Their combined effects have led to a disruption and weakening of the conventional family-based model (Dhemba & Dhemba, 2015). This means that, in certain cases, instead of the younger generation including children and grandchildren caring for older adults, the reverse is becoming more common (Makiwane et al., 2022). That is, in addition to the personal issues that older people face such as the decline in the functional ability, they must also care for children and grandchildren who have been orphaned by HIV/AIDS or whose parents have moved in search of opportunities elsewhere (Munthree & Maharaj, 2010; Dhemba & Dhemba, 2015; Noyoo, 2017). In most cases, the grandmother takes on most of the burden of caregiving responsibilities for their children and grandchildren. This informal caregiving takes place in the context of widespread poverty, limited support, stigma, and accusations of witchcraft as well as many of the other challenges frequently facing people in their old age (Kulu & Hannemann, 2016).

In many households, older adults assume different roles other than household headship. Studies highlight the significance of grandparents in offering care to children living within their households, both material and financial support (Kulu & Hannemann, 2016; Schatz & Ogunmefun, 2007). Grandparents have a wealth of knowledge and expertise that they instil in the younger generation. They often are the ones who support their grandchildren, provide stability and faith, and whom everyone looks to when life tosses unexpected obstacles (Makiwane et al., 2022). In addition, grandparents play a crucial role in preserving and fostering traditional values and beliefs. Furthermore, many family members look to their grandparents for guidance. In traditional societies, grandparents frequently had a direct and visible role in the care and development of children. Urbanisation has made it necessary for older adults to also look after younger family members while their parents move to other areas in search of work opportunities. When mothers leave, grandparents assume the responsibility for their grandchildren. This is particularly true for older women who tend to take it upon themselves to provide much of the care in their households (Schatz et al., 2018). Baloyi (2015) contends that in South Africa, older adults are frequently forced to use their old age grants or pensions to support their grandchildren. Childcare arrangements are an important consideration that can impact a mother's decision to relocate and begin working. For many mothers with young children, employment is dictated by geographical access to childcare facilities, but a lack of such facilities does not impede a mother's move because grandparents frequently fill this function (Majola et al., 2023).

There are few formal care systems in sub-Saharan Africa, particularly in South Africa outside of the health sector; instead, families care for children, the sick, and the elderly (Apt, 2012). South Africa is among the many nations that encourage older adults to live as long as possible in community settings due to the excessive costs associated with institutional elderly care provision (Billings & Leichsenring, 2007). Multigenerational households are frequently the focus of care work that includes financial, instrumental, emotional, and psychosocial support for both older adults and their family members (Schatz et al., 2018). Furthermore, multigenerational networks help the elderly and children under their care by promoting their wellbeing (Schatz et al., 2018). Children's wellbeing in such situations depends on both immediate family resources and extended kin networks (Apt, 2012), including grandmothers and aunts, but also grandfathers and uncles, frequently contribute significantly to children's diverse needs. The older people, who are beneficiaries of the means-tested, non-contributory old age pension for men and women aged 60 years and older, frequently contribute the only income in their households due to the high rate of unemployment in South Africa; as a result, they must sustain their entire family solely on their old age grant stipend (Potts, 2012). The pension may be used to lessen the financial burden by making sure that the grandchildren within the household have access to food, clothing, shelter, education, and other necessities (Sekhampu & Grobler, 2011). The presence or absence of support or resources, as well as the need for older adults to care for others, can either accommodate or exacerbate their health conditions (Samanta et al., 2015; Nyirenda et al., 2015). Until recently much of the focus on older people has been on the care that they provide to their children and grandchildren. However, there has been little attention paid to the reciprocity that exists in these relationships. The focus of this chapter is to understand the lived experiences of older people in providing and receiving care.

Researching Older People in a Township

To gain an insider perspective into the experiences of older people, this study employed a qualitative approach drawing on 20 face-to-face semi-structured interviews. The interviews explore how older people navigate the difficult and precarious socio-economic situation in which they are living. Interviews were conducted with older men and women in KwaNdengezi township. The apartheid government built residences for Black communities who were relocated to townships under the Group Areas Act. KwaNdengezi is situated in KwaZulu-Natal, South Africa's second most populous province. The township has approximately 54,000 residents (Gumede & Napier, 2022).

The size of the sample was determined by the availability of willing participants. Some were not willing to participate in the study because they did not want to speak to strangers. In order to be eligible for the study, men and women had to be aged 60 years and older. After identifying the initial participants, snowball sampling was utilised to identify other potential participants with similar characteristics. The interviews were conducted by researchers trained in qualitative data collecting techniques. Given the cultural expectations of courtesy and respect when interacting with older adults, the interviewers were from the area and shared the same cultural background with the participants to avoid any misunderstandings that could distort the data. All the interviews were conducted in the homesteads of participants or in spaces they identified for their privacy and comfort. Each interview lasted on average 40 minutes. All interviews were done in isiZulu, the language spoken by most people in KwaNdengezi township. After consent was sought and given, all the interviews were digitally recorded and later translated and transcribed into English. Confidentiality and anonymity were strictly observed. To ensure that the identity of the 20 participants is protected, no real names of participants are used in this chapter. Additionally, the researchers ensured that informed consent was granted from all study participants. The interviewers explained to the participants that the information they shared was going to be kept strictly confidential and used only for academic purposes. Consent was sought and granted prior to recording all the interviews. The interview transcripts were analysed using the thematic analysis method. The transcripts were read and then sorted based on emerging themes. However, rather than focusing just on common themes, consideration was given to how well it aligned with the study's aims.

The age of the interviewed participants ranged from 60 to 78 years. The educational levels varied, with some only completing their primary schooling, others having some secondary education, and only one participant having a college certificate. The majority were unemployed, with only one employed and the other was self-employed. As people age, they are more likely to be married. Among the interviewed participants, seven were married, one was widowed, and the remaining were single. All participants reported that they had at least one child. Moreover, the participants came from homes that have between three to eight household members. All the participants were residents of KwaNdengezi township, and all were also recipients of the old age grant offered by the government as a means to alleviate poverty among the population.

Deterioration in Their Health

As people age, their health declines. Almost all the participants stated that they were experiencing health problems. The most common health conditions included diabetes, arthritis, high blood pressure, and hypertension. Others reported that while they were not suffering from a specific sickness, they noticed that their health had deteriorated over time. They believed that they had become progressively weaker physically over the past few years because of stressors in their homes, which had rapidly brought about their illness.

> "I have high blood pressure, I am diabetic, and minor symptoms of arthritis although I have not yet begun to treat it. I am diabetic, I have BP [hypertension], and spinal cord arthritis. I am undergoing treatment for it at Chief Albert Luthuli Hospital and at RK Khan Hospital".

It is apparent that older adults tend to suffer mostly from non-communicable diseases that are detrimental to their lives. This indicates that as people age, they require more care and support to alleviate their health burden, which might otherwise aggravate their condition. The care provided to older adults would shield them from stressors that would contribute to further deterioration in their health.

Accessing Health Care

As people age there is a greater demand for health care. All South Africans, inclusive of older adults, are entitled to free public primary healthcare services. However, many encounter barriers to proper care and support, and they may underutilise or receive insufficient care. When the participants were questioned about accessing healthcare services, their responses varied with most accessing free state-owned healthcare services.

> "I go to our local clinic [KwaNdengezi clinic]. Also, my son-in-law has medical aid. So, they would sometimes take me to a private hospital, but this is usually when I am seriously ill, if its minor sicknesses I go to our local clinic".

> "Yes, unless the doctor advice otherwise. Also, this is a government hospital, you are not guaranteed to see the same doctor every time you visit. They would alternate".

Some concern was expressed about the lack of continuity of services in public health facilities. One older man highlighted that in government hospitals or clinics they are not seen by the same doctor on every visit, suggesting that the medical staff may not have established a relationship with the older person. In this case, there is a lower likelihood of continuity in care.

Some older people also utilise private health facilities but are only able to do so because they are receiving support from their children. One older woman explained that her children pay for her to access healthcare services when the need arises. Children play an important role in taking care of the health care needs of their parents, especially if they can afford it.

> "I access health care through a private health practitioner and my children pay cash. They are really good at taking care of me. I remember when my other son was still alive, I would not even pay for electricity, he would do everything for me. He would say here is cash or go to a certain place I left some money for you".

Even though healthcare services are offered free of charge in South Africa, the monetary costs and the time spent travelling to a health facility represents out of pocket cost of accessing healthcare. These expenditures may present a considerable barrier for vulnerable segments of the population such as older adults, resulting in overall poor health. Family members are instrumental in assisting older adults in accessing healthcare services, especially if they are in a position to provide financial support. However, older adults may also feel reluctant to burden their family members with their problems. In addition, they want to remain self-sufficient and independent.

All the interviewed participants for this study did not cite travelling costs to and from healthcare facilities as a barrier to accessing these facilities. When questioned about how they travel to and from healthcare facilities some participants cited that they walk as the facilities are in close proximity to their place of residence. However, they indicated that they would receive support from family members to get to a health facility if the need arose.

> "I walk but sometimes I use my son's car when he is available, I just tell them to take me there. But if there is no car, I am always happy to walk because it is not that far".

> "It is R20 for a return trip, so it is too little, I pay for it and our clinic is a free service clinic".

Some participants also use public transportation whenever the need for them to access healthcare services arises. They felt that this was the most convenient form of transportation available to them. In addition, they observed that the travelling costs are not too exorbitant, so they are able to afford it. The interviews revealed that older adults do not want to burden their children unless absolutely necessary. They draw on their own resources, such as pensions and savings, before turning to their children for support. While this is commendable, older adults tend to incur out-of-pocket costs which are not reimbursed. Studies on the effects of out-of-pocket costs for older adults experiencing particular health conditions indicate that spending associated with these conditions affects their capacity to pay for necessities such as food (Piette et al., 2004; Essue et al., 2011).

Recognising the Need for Care for Themselves

With an increasing life expectancy comes a greater reliance on others for care. This was no different to the study's participants who felt that as they grow older more emphasis should be on care provision. The provision of care to the older population would go a long way in ensuring that they live happy lives. When participants were asked if they need to be taken care of, most of them agreed, observing that they no longer have the physical strength to do things on their own as they used to in their youthful years.

> "Yes, always. As you can see. I do everything in this house because there is no other way. If I had the means, I would hire a helper to help me with collecting my medication, with the house chores and taking care of my grandchildren".

> "Yes, it happens that I am not able to do things for myself. Sometimes I cannot walk so I do need someone to take care of me".

> "Yes, sometimes I do feel like I need someone to take care of me, massage me when I am not feeling okay, or just pamper me".

As people age, they tend to lose their physical strength and are no longer able to do the things they could in their youth. Older adults need maximum care as they are among the most vulnerable members of society. Support for older adults in the form of instrumental aid and emotional comfort helps to relieve stress, lessen depressive symptoms, and minimise the negative health impacts of stressful life events (Croezen et al., 2012). In the interviews, some older adults admitted that they experienced difficulties carrying out household activities and they needed assistance and even care. They recognised their frailty as a barrier to their full participation in activities of daily living as they experienced challenges when doing household chores. For them, care provision would go a long way in assisting them with the activities of daily living. The ideal situation would be to hire someone to take care of their needs but for the vast majority this is not an option as they do not have the funds, as they are reliant on their old age pension.

> "Yes, sometimes I do feel I need to be taken care of because in my current age I am no longer able to do things I could in the past. I mean things that require strength such as cooking, washing of cloths and sometimes cleaning".

> "Yes, sometimes I do see the need to be taken care of. My child, I tend to get tired, cooking, cleaning every day and doing other things in the house is tiring. I feel like I need someone who can do all these things for me".

Care provision is especially important in the lives of the elderly. The quality of life and health outcomes for older adults are improved by greater social networks, or the connections between groups of familiar people and the care provided to them. As a result, care provision for older people is identified as crucial for a high quality of life. The absence of significant care provision and social connections also causes older adults to retreat from their social networks. While the lack of adequate care provision is a risk factor for increased illness susceptibility and mortality, it is also a predictor of disease outcomes for older people, resulting in a lower quality of life (Khan & Tahir, 2014). When participants were asked about disabilities pertaining to their daily functioning, most of them highlighted that they could do basic things such as bathing themselves, going to the toilet, and making food, but they admitted that they experienced challenges with doing household chores. Some stated that they are cautious about their health, so in mitigating the risk they hire people to assist them with household chores but this is only an option for the few.

> "Yes, I am able to do basic things on my own such as bathing, going to the toilet and making food".

> "We sometimes get a helper to assist with most of the work because arthritis and cold water can send you straight to hospital. Our helper would do the washing and cleaning the house and the rest we take care of it".

Some participants highlighted that they experience mobility problems but try and maintain their independence. They noted that since they live in houses with stairs, they sometimes battle to get to some areas in their homes. This can be linked to functional disability, because as people age, they tend to witness a deterioration when it comes to functionality. In this case, the support from other family members is very valuable. In most cases, the grandchildren tend to serve as carers and offer them assistance, whenever the need arises.

> "Most of the time when I am sick, I tend to battle with climbing the stairs, but my grandchildren are always assisting in such instances. But I can do everything else on my own. I don't need help".

> "My knees are painful so I cannot even climb stairs. They [doctors] once said I will have an operation, the next thing they said I am too old for it. So, I find it difficult to walk. You would think I am an old granny!".

For most older people, mobility impairments placed the most restrictions on them. Because of this, they had to rely on others for assistance in carrying out activities of daily living. The most frequent source of assistance was other family members including a spouse or child. However, a few reported not receiving any care or support. Physical support from sources external to the family was limited, with only one saying that they relied on paid help. Living with family has been linked to greater health for older people as well as greater social support and care (Hosegood & Timaeus, 2005). Care and support are fundamental elements for older people, as they are at high-risk for anxiety. Moreover, physical functions gradually deteriorate as they age, and the impact of social role shifts, the loss of loved ones and other adverse events can induce anxiety in older adults. As people age, they are also more prone to functional disability which vastly hinders them from doing any household chores. This responsibility is usually filled by their children along with grandchildren.

When the participants were questioned about the availability of care and support from within their households, some indicated that they deal with household chores themselves but admitted that they do receive support from their families as well. They did not want to see themselves as a burden to their family. Older adults prefer to maintain their independence and autonomy, and only turn to their children and grandchildren when they have limited options available, a finding consistent with another study in South Africa (Rabie & Klopper, 2015). In many households, older adults bear the responsibility of having to care for family members. As they spend most of their time at home, they feel happier when they are busy with the day-to-day household duties. Some participants stated that they rotate household duties with their family members, in that way everyone bears the responsibility of care provision within the households. Most wanted to remain active so they assist in household chores.

> "I do the washing, cooking, and cleaning. We alternate, sometimes my son would clean the house, my grandson would wash his clothes and I would cook. In this house, everyone washes their clothes and sometimes they would clean. When it comes to cooking, I cook".

Providing Care to Others

It is not uncommon for older people to live in multigenerational households with their children and grandchildren. Multigenerational households that include children, parents, and grandparents, irrespective of whether they are biologically related or not, are mostly the locus of care work for old and young (Schatz et al., 2018), promoting their wellbeing.

Older people play an important role in the lives of their children. They often assume the responsibility of caregiving to their grandchildren. They attend to all the care needs of their grandchildren including other youth within their households. Participants shared varied experiences pertaining to care provision within their homes and communities; highlighting their day-to-day lived experiences of caregiving. Older people frequently take on many household chores to ease the burden on other members. As caregivers to grandchildren and other family members who need care, older people tend to prioritise basic household tasks such as ironing of school clothes, preparing food, and attending to all basic care needs of their family members.

> "Yes, there is my granddaughter. I wake up in the morning and prepare for school, make her lunch box, iron her clothes and when she comes back from school, I have to prepare food for her".

Older people frequently provide care to immediate family members such as grandchildren and other youth, which has been brought on by lack of employment opportunities nearby. Often their children are forced to move and seek opportunities elsewhere and when this happens, the grandparents are left with their grandchildren. This means that their grandchildren not only live with them but they also have to take full responsibility for the care of them.

According to Statistics South Africa (2024) quarterly labour statistics, youth unemployment stands at 59.4%. This denotes that a huge proportion of the youth is unemployed. The high unemployment among their children has a negative impact on older people because it results in them having to bear the brunt of providing care within their households. This is a major cause of stress that might impact older people's health negatively.

> "I am not happy because there is no way forward for us. I mean my son is unemployed. If he finds a job, these days jobs are only temporary. So, for me life is at a standstill. I am grateful for having a home but life inside these walls is a struggle".

It is evident that outside of the health sector, older people frequently nurture and care for others within their households. One woman indicated that she cares for a relative who can no longer walk: *"Yes, we have a relative, she cannot walk anymore, and I have to care for her as she cannot do most things on her own"*. Some participants observed that they do not have a choice when it comes to providing care to some family members such as grandchildren and those who are sick. One woman explained: *"It's not like I have a choice, my grandchildren are my responsibility"*. Older people do not only care for only close family members but extend care to people within their communities who need care. This is because some people within their communities do not have immediate family members who would provide care to them, hence they step in to provide support for those requiring assistance within their communities.

> "Yes, she (my sister) is also diabetic. Her sugar levels are very high, she needs injections. I take care of her".

> "There is another elderly woman who had a stroke, so I had to take her to the hospital with the bill on me and she was not the first one, I always help people who are sick".

Older people are a valuable source of care provision not only for their family members but also the wider community. Some feel that they are left with no choice because they are the only ones with the means to provide care within their homes and sometimes communities. All the older people were recipients of the state-sponsored old age pension. Sometimes they are faced with limited resources, but they have little option but to use it to care for those who are in need, particularly their immediate family members.

The main source of income for older adults is the old age pension. Older adults acknowledge that most of their pension is used to cover their household monthly expenses. When the participants were questioned how they utilise their social support grant within their households it was clear that many households are dependent on their pension for their monthly expenses.

> "Because I have to pay for the water bill, buy prepaid electricity, and buy groceries but my children sometimes buy food when they have some money".

> "I sometimes buy groceries, buy electricity and use it to cover my travelling expenses when I need to visit the clinic".

Older people are dependent on their pension for their survival. They reported utilising their old age grants to cover the basic necessities in the household. Some of the necessities include paying for groceries, electricity, and water accounts, along with transport costs to and from the health care facilities. Only one participant is able to utilise her old age grant to cater for her own needs. According to her, *"I do my personal stuff, like buying cosmetics, I use my money to have fun and enjoy myself"*. She does not have to take responsibilities for major expenses like water, and electricity within her household. She was one of the few who was able to use her grant to meet her own needs and that was because her children were employed and able to support her.

It is important to note that the harsh economic situation in the country affects all the citizens including older adults, who often shoulder the responsibility of providing for the family sometimes with their old age grant. As populations age, they are likely to face a number of issues that have a negative impact on their lived experiences within their households. The most obvious issues raised by the participants were largely economic in nature. The older people also mentioned how, as pensioners, they frequently struggle to pay their bills. Older people struggle to make ends meet within their households as they are mostly responsible for covering the basic services. They highlighted the high cost of electricity and water, stating that a huge chunk of their old age social grant goes to paying off these services. Sometimes they are faced with difficult choices about how they spend their pension and this puts enormous pressure on their ability to make ends meet.

Conclusion

Ageing in South Africa is occurring in the context of high levels of poverty, inequality, and unemployment as well as an increasing burden of communicable and non-communicable health conditions. A person's environment, and those within it, have a direct social effect on how care and support is reciprocated. As people get older their health begins to decline and they may need assistance to carry out the activities of daily living. Older people are dependent on family members for support and care but they also provide care and support to others, particularly for young members of their households. In many households, the old age pension is the only source of income and therefore provides valuable financial support especially in the context of high youth unemployment. This is likely to influence the way older people are perceived and treated. What is clear is that older people perform important functions and the relationship is not one directional.

References

Apt, N. A. (2012). Aging in Africa: Past experiences and strategic directions. *Ageing International, 37*(1), 93–103.

Baloyi, M. E. (2015). A pastoral investigation into some of the challenges associated with aging and retirement in the South African context. *In die Skriflig, 49*(3), 1–10.

Bengtson, V. L., & Martin, P. (2001). Families and intergenerational relationships in aging societies: Comparing the United States with German-speaking countries. *Zeitschrift für Gerontologie und Geriatrie, 34*, 207–217.

Billings, J., & Leichsenring, K. (Eds.). (2007). *Integrating health and social care services for older persons: Evidence from nine European countries*. Ashgate.

Croezen, S., Picavet, S. J., Haveman-Nies, A., Verschuren, W. M., De Groot, L., & Veer, P. (2012). Do positive or negative experiences of social support relate to current and future health? Results from the Doetinchem cohort study. *BMC Public Health, 12*, 65.

Dhemba, J., & Dhemba, B. (2015). Ageing and care of older persons in Southern Africa: Lesotho and Zimbabwe compared. *Social Work & Society, 13*(2), 1–16.

Essue, B., Kelly, P., Roberts, M., Leeder, S., & Jan, S. (2011). We can't afford my chronic illness! The out-of-pocket burden associated with managing chronic obstructive pulmonary disease in western Sydney, Australia. *Journal of Health Services Research & Policy, 16*(4), 226–231.

Gumede, C., & Napier, S. (2022). Food consumption patterns, socio-demographic status, and nutritional risks of women in low- and middle-income communities in Kwandengezi, Kwazulu-Natal, South Africa. *African Journal of Food, Agriculture, Nutrition and Development, 22*(4), 20121–20147.

Hosegood, V., & Timeaus, I. (2005). The impact of adult mortality on the living arrangements of older people in rural South Africa. *Ageing & Society, 25*(6), 431–444.

Kengne, A. P., & Mayosi, B. M. (2014). Readiness of the primary care system for non-communicable diseases in sub-Saharan Africa. *The Lancet Global Health, 2*(5), 247–248.

Khan, A. R., & Tahir, I. (2014). Influence of social factors to the quality of life of the elderly in Malaysia. *Open Medicine Journal, 1*(1), 29.

Kulu, H., & Hannemann, T. (2016). Introduction to research on immigrant and ethnic minority families in Europe. *Demographic Research, 35*(2), 31–46.

Lehohla, P. (2014). *Census 2011: Profile of older persons in South Africa.* Statistics South Africa.

Majola, T., Dunn, S., & Maharaj, P. (2023). Childcare arrangements of migrant mothers in an urban township in South Africa. *Gender, Place & Culture, 30*(1), 92–110.

Makiwane, M., Alubafi, M. F., & Gumede, N. A. (2022). Understanding and evaluating older persons services: The case of the Gauteng Province, South Africa. *Journal of Population Ageing, 15*(4), 999–1015.

Munthree, C., & Maharaj, P. (2010). Growing old in the era of a high prevalence of HIV/AIDS: The impact of AIDS on older men and women in KwaZulu-Natal, South Africa. *Research on Aging, 32*(2), 155–174.

Noyoo, N. (2017). Reflecting on the human rights of older persons in South Africa. *Journal of Human Rights and Social Work, 2*(4), 108–116.

Nyirenda, M., Evandrou, M., Mutevedzi, P., Hosegood, V., Falkingham, J., & Newell, M. L. (2015). Who cares? Implications of caregiving and-receiving by HIV-infected or-affected older people on functional disability and emotional wellbeing. *Ageing & Society, 35*(1), 169–202.

Piette, J. D., Heisler, M., & Wagner, T. H. (2004). Problems paying out-of-pocket medication costs among older adults with diabetes. *Diabetes Care, 27*(2), 384–391.

Potts, R. (2012). Social welfare in South Africa: Curing or causing poverty. *Penn State Journal of International Affairs, 2*(1), 74–92.
Rabie, T., & Klopper, H. C. (2015). Guidelines to facilitate self-care among older persons in South Africa. *Health SA Gesondheid, 20*(1), 33–34.
Samanta, T., Chen, F., & Vanneman, R. (2015). Living arrangements and health of older adults in India. *Journals of Gerontology Series B: Psychological Sciences and Social Sciences, 70*(6), 937–947.
Schatz, E., & Ogunmefun, C. (2007). Caring and contributing: The role of older women in rural south African multi-generational households in the HIV/AIDA era. *World Development, 35*(8), 1390–1403.
Schatz, E., Seeley, J., & Zalwango, F. (2018). Intergenerational care for and by children: Examining reciprocity through focus group interviews with older adults in rural Uganda. *Demographic Research, 38*(63), 2003–2026.
Sekhampu, T. J., & Grobler, W. (2011). The expenditure patterns of households receiving the State's Old Age Pension (SOAP) grant in Kwakwatsi Township. *The Journal for Transdisciplinary Research in Southern Africa, 7*(1), 41–52.
Statistics South Africa. (2024). *Quarterly labour force survey 2024.*
Świderska, M. (2014). The importance of family support in old age. *Pedagogika Rodziny, 4*(1), 15–22.
Thomas, P. A., Liu, H., & Umberson, D. (2017). Family relationships and well-being. *Innovation in Aging, 1*(3), igx025.
Wang, L., Yang, L., Di, X., & Dai, X. (2020). Family support, multidimensional health, and living satisfaction among the elderly: A case from Shaanxi Province, China. *International Journal of Environmental Research and Public Health, 17*(22), 8434.
World Health Organization (WHO). (2002). *Active ageing. A policy framework.* World Health Organization.
World Health Organization (WHO). (2015a). *The growing need for home health care for the elderly: Home health care for the elderly as an integral part of primary health care services.* World Health Organization.
World Health Organization (WHO). (2015b). *Ageing and health.* World Health Organization.
World Health Organization (WHO). (2015c). *Global action plan for the prevention and control of noncommunicable diseases 2013–2020.* World Health Organization.

7

"I Would Never Be Able to Pay If It Was Not for My Children": A Qualitative Study of Obstacles Facing Older People in Obtaining Healthcare

Sachin Sewpersad and Pranitha Maharaj

Abstract South Africa's healthcare system is already under a great deal of pressure, and the increasing population of elderly is expected to exacerbate the many challenges already experienced by healthcare services. Among older Indians, chronic illnesses such as diabetes and hypertension are among the leading causes of mortality in South Africa. To better understand experiences in accessing healthcare services, this study draws on 20 in-depth interviews with older Indian men and women. The interviews revealed that older Indian adults face various barriers to accessing healthcare services, ranging from physical and functional challenges, to transportation and poverty. They often rely on their children to pay for their medical insurance, or they provide them with transportation to receive healthcare. Older adults lean on family for support and assistance in meeting their healthcare needs. However, given the magnitude of the healthcare needs of older people, family can no longer support them alone.

S. Sewpersad (✉) • P. Maharaj
School of Built Environment and Development Studies, University of KwaZulu-Natal, Durban, South Africa
e-mail: SewpersadS@ukzn.ac.za; Maharajp7@ukzn.ac.za

P. Maharaj (ed.), *Navigating Ageing in South Africa*, Sustainable Development Goals Series, https://doi.org/10.1007/978-981-97-9088-3_7

Keywords Healthcare needs • Ageing • Access • Utilisation • Indians • South Africa

Introduction

Like many other countries around the world, South Africa is currently witnessing a growth in the number of older people. The country has one of the most rapidly ageing populations in Africa, and older people constitute an ever-increasing share of the population. Currently, persons aged 60 years and older constitute approximately 9% (or 5.5 million) of the total population of the country (Statistics South Africa, 2022). However, over the next decade, the number of people aged 60 years and over is expected to increase. It is estimated that by 2030, South Africa would already have around 15 million older people (Kelly et al., 2019). This is likely to create an increase in dependency and place more pressure on support systems for older people, particularly health services.

While older people are living longer, it is often in poor health. As people age, they are at higher risk of developing chronic non-communicable health conditions, such as cardiovascular diseases, chronic respiratory diseases, hypertension, and diabetes (Adhikari & Rijal, 2014). In addition, communicable diseases such as HIV are also common among older people, especially in South Africa (Aboderin & Beard, 2015). Older people are particularly vulnerable to emerging diseases such as COVID-19 and face an elevated risk of contracting severe infections due to the numerous potential underlying health conditions that they already suffer from (WHO, 2020). Older people in less developed countries are also particularly vulnerable to short-term illnesses due to high levels of infection and poor living conditions. These diseases include lower respiratory infections, diarrheal diseases, and malaria (Streatfield et al., 2014; Troeger et al., 2018).

The health system is already under a great deal of pressure, and the increasing population of elderly is expected to exacerbate the many challenges already experienced by healthcare services. Local clinics and health centres are the primary entry point into the healthcare system where people are initially treated, whilst emergency cases are referred to the district hospital, which is the secondary level of care (Ameh et al., 2014). Healthcare is divided into a publicly funded system that serves the majority of the population and a privately funded system that serves the minority of people who are able to afford it (Kon & Lackan, 2008). There is also rivalry between both sectors, as medical professionals prefer to work in the more profitable private sector (Kon & Lackan, 2008). However, the choice of healthcare service provider in South Africa is increasingly dominated by economic factors. There is a general dissatisfaction with public sector health services with some of the reasons being the non-availability of prescribed medication, poor attitude of staff, and long waiting periods (Hasumi & Jacobsen, 2014; Sekhejane, 2013). In contrast, the private health service has many advantages such as shorter waiting times, unrushed appointments, better facilities, and proper disease control and prevention practices. Those who use private facilities also experience some dissatisfaction; however, these are usually related to finances and cost (Hasumi & Jacobsen, 2014), especially among those who cannot afford medical aid or private care.

South Africa is one of the most unequal societies in the world, and this is largely a legacy of apartheid's discriminatory and racially biased policies. The apartheid system of separation resulted in unequal access to infrastructure and services among certain groups who were also situated in geographically disadvantaged areas (Mtapuri & Tinarwo, 2021). Apartheid policies also resulted in a 'fragmented and discriminatory health service' (Maharaj & Cleland, 2005: p. 311) with extreme variations in the quality and accessibility of services depending on place of residence and racial group (Maphumulo & Bhengu, 2019). This resulted in the deterioration in the health system due to the lack of resources, and poor communities were particularly affected (Chassin & Loeb, 2013).

Poverty is highly prevalent and a major barrier to accessing healthcare for the elderly. The costs of chronic diseases are continuously increasing and are a major public health burden (Liu et al., 2015). Poverty deters health-seeking behaviour as the elderly consider seeking treatment for their illnesses to be a waste of money (Adhikari & Rijal, 2014). Out-of-pocket spending on healthcare may further exacerbate the financial problems already faced by the elderly who depend on social grants for an income (Dokpesi, 2017). Poverty therefore causes unequal access to healthcare resources and also affects other basic needs of the elderly, such as access to clean water, sanitation, nutritious food, housing and shelter, education, and overall quality of life (Wandera et al., 2015).

Some elderly also put their faith in religion to heal them of diseases and ailments and believe that medical care is not required, which may only seek to exacerbate their conditions (Adhikari & Rijal, 2014). There are sometimes negative perceptions of 'Western' medications and treatments, as some believe that they are detrimental if taken in excess and therefore incorrectly self-adjust their medication dosage (Zeh et al., 2014). Women seem to be more restricted by cultural barriers due to the fear of physical harassment, gender norms, and socio-cultural rules and expectations that oppress and prevent them from visiting health services (Zeh et al., 2014). Women's access to healthcare is also limited by traditional beliefs and culture, especially since they have multiple roles in society and in their households, which require them to prioritise the needs of men and children over themselves (Aboyade et al., 2016). Traditionally, elders were respected in society; however, changing times and modernism have eroded these cultural norms, resulting in the abuse and neglect of the elderly (Bigala & Ayiga, 2014). Other cultural challenges include the belief that poor health is just another part of ageing and getting older, and this is a major deterrent to seeking healthcare (Adhikari & Rijal, 2014).

Distance poses a major barrier to accessing healthcare. High transport costs, especially to health facilities, may dissuade health-seeking behaviour for prompt treatment. Without transport, it is very difficult for the elderly to travel to health facilities, especially those with disabilities, frailties, and other elements that prevent them from walking long distances (Aboyade et al., 2016). Lack of transportation may also cause missed appointments with doctors or delayed treatment and therefore consistency in the management of non-communicable diseases (Syed et al., 2013). Aboyade et al. (2016) state that non-communicable diseases are poorly managed in Africa due to infrequent access, caused by the lack of transport, to the required health facility to obtain medication. Long distances to health facilities limit access to health (Maharaj, 2013) and may also interrupt chronic treatment for ailments such as HIV.

Although health is a major concern for all age groups, to date, limited empirical research has been conducted in many developing countries on the older population. Additionally, there are few studies conducted among minorities, particularly Indians in South Africa. Existing literature suggests a growing body of evidence on the situation of older people, but there is a noticeable dearth of information on older Indians. This may result in severe inequalities in policy and intervention formulation. Therefore, this sort of challenge must be addressed to allow minorities to participate in society, politics, and the economy.

Focus on Older Indians

Indians constitute almost 1.5 million or 2.6% of the country's total population, forming one of the major population groups in South Africa (Statistics South Africa, 2021). Indians in South Africa also have a high ageing rate (Statistics South Africa, 2014), indicating the need for more research on older people in this group. Even though Indians have had a strong presence in South Africa for well over 150 years and are officially recognised as one of the major population groups, they have not been the focus of much research. The small size of the population has ultimately resulted in their neglect in many studies, especially with regard to ageing. The aim of this chapter is to fill this gap by focusing on the health-seeking behaviour of older Indians in Durban, South Africa.

Studies suggest that chronic illnesses such as diabetes and hypertension are some of the leading causes of mortality in South Africa and are highly prevalent among Indians in the country (Prabhakaran et al., 2016; Prakaschandra et al., 2016). A study by Prakaschandra et al. (2016) was the first to document the dangerously high prevalence of cardiovascular diseases among Indians. The study explains that these diseases are highly prevalent in this population group and their rates of change over the past few decades have been of epidemic proportions (Prakaschandra et al., 2016). This is a major cause for concern, especially in light of the ongoing coronavirus pandemic, as these chronic illnesses significantly increase the risk of complications and mortality from infections, especially in older persons (Zhou et al., 2020).

Many Indians arrived in South Africa during the colonial era as indentured labourers to work in the agricultural sector and were also subjected to the tyranny of apartheid. Durban still faces issues pertaining to reconciliation on a daily basis, as the city was formerly segregated along racial lines as part of the Group Areas Act during the apartheid era, a period in which society was explicitly and systemically racially segregated (Seekings, 2008). Residential areas were racially segregated, and this marginalised the poorer residents of the city, creating geographic barriers to accessing resources such as education and health services (Schoeman, 2018). The Group Areas Act of 1950, one of the main legal instruments used to reinforce apartheid, divided towns and cities of South Africa by race. This study was conducted in a suburb, Avoca, which historically mainly consisted of Indians. Avoca was chosen as the study site due to the large number of older Indians living in the area.

Geographically, Avoca is north of the city centre, and is situated in a hilly region, with a network of rivers and streams intersecting parts of the area. The suburb has a lot of greenery and open spaces for recreational purposes and is mainly a residential area; however, there are also a few light industries. Avoca is highly accessible by road and railway and is a relatively well-developed area with brick houses, and proper sanitation and water supply. In terms of socio-economic background, the suburb is described as a middle-income area. The suburb has many landmarks owing to the strong presence of the Indians, including religious places of worship and memorials.

The qualitative data for the study comes from 20 in-depth interviews with Indian men and women aged 60 years and older. A number of strategies were used to recruit older people for the study, including directly approaching them and asking for referrals to other potential participants. The strategies used ensured that the sample constituted a range of older people. Qualitative methods were best suited for identifying the range of factors that influence health behaviour. An interview schedule was used to guide the data collection, and interviews began by obtaining socio-economic and demographic information. The guide covered a range of topics, including health status, choices about healthcare, and challenges in obtaining health services.

The average age of participants was 67 years old, with the youngest aged 60 and the oldest aged 80. Five of the 20 participants were male, and the remaining 15 were female. Level of education was relatively high with the majority having obtained at least some secondary education. One participant was unable to recall their highest level of education. The majority were married at some point in time, but only seven participants were currently married. All the married participants were living with their spouses. In the sample, there was only one person who had never married. The remaining were previously married but, at the time of the interviews, were either divorced or widowed. Of the 20 participants, only three lived alone with the remaining living with other family members including their spouse and children. All participants were living in the area for many years, and all were receiving the old-age social grant. In the sample, four participants were employed at the time of the interview.

The interviews took place over a three-month period. All the interviews were conducted by the first author, an Indian male living in the community. This was useful in establishing rapport with the participants and ensuring rich detailed descriptions in the interviews. Each interview was conducted in English and lasted on average one hour. The venue, in most cases, was their place of residence, which was the most convenient location for the participants and ensured maximum privacy. At all times, there was a strong emphasis on confidentiality. Participation in the study was voluntary, and participants were free to withdraw at any time after having signed the informed consent form or giving verbal consent.

Ethical approval for the study was obtained from the University of KwaZulu-Natal. All the interviews were digitally recorded and later transcribed. The interviews were analysed using thematic analysis. The data was categorised into a number of themes and then initial codes or labels were applied to segments of the data. Salient themes in the interviews were identified and used to form a coding framework. The coding framework assisted in the analysis to make comparisons.

Living with Sickness

Ageing is often accompanied by multiple and severe chronic illnesses. The lives of many older people are dominated by chronic illnesses which are usually accompanied by functional and physical limitations that negatively impact their quality of life. As people age, they are also more likely to experience multi-morbidities that may lead to negative interactions between each condition or their specific treatments. In addition, multi-morbidities are associated with higher usage of health services which also increases the pressure on health systems as populations age (Bähler et al., 2015).

In the interviews, it became clear that sickness is a daily reality for many older adults. They suffer from a range of chronic health problems, including hypertension, diabetes, cardiovascular diseases, high cholesterol, and thyroid disorders. Men and women also complained of debilitating chronic pain which affected their mobility and limited their functional ability to perform daily activities of living. They spoke of '*tiredness*', '*shortness of breath*', '*headaches*', '*legs that do not always function*', '*weakness in feet*', '*pain in knees*', and '*suffering*'. Chronic health conditions require medication that must be taken lifelong, and since older people are likely to have to live with more than one of these chronic diseases, they must take several types of medication on a daily basis. In some cases, they experience difficulties in maintaining normal body functions such as walking, eating, and bathing.

> "I had cancer of the colon. In 2016, I had heart triple bypass. I got spine problems, and diabetes. I also suffer from rheumatic arthritis; my legs do not always function. I feel weak on my feet on my own, like I cannot walk on my own. If I go anywhere, I have somebody to hold me" (Nisha, 78 years).

> "I am suffering with pain in my knees on my two legs and I get severe headaches so I am taking my treatment in hospital" (Katherine, 64 years).

> "It is sad because you are not able to do the things you used to do like walk briskly from one place to another, and when you slow down you seem to be in the way of other people who are moving much faster than you are" (Freya, 69 years).

As their health deteriorates and the prevalence of disabilities, cognitive decline and frailty increases, older people may lose independence and thus require support (Ralston et al., 2016; Ren & Treiman, 2015; Schatz et al., 2015). In the interviews, it was clear that autonomy may be severely constrained by illness and older people may find themselves having to depend more heavily on others for support. A few older people with more serious ailments reported that they require more care and attention, often from family members. It was also not uncommon to find that some older people suffer from several health complications. Men and women with chronic conditions require specialised health services. They also have to visit a health facility at least once a month for a routine examination and also to obtain their medication.

Most older people, despite having several chronic health conditions, displayed a positive attitude towards living. They displayed an understanding that ageing is often accompanied by poor health. There was an acceptance of their health situation and the deterioration in health because of their age.

> "I feel like we must not lose hope, you know, even if we got aches and pains, continue with life. Life goes on!" (Anna, 67).

> "Well, there is nothing much to say because, I mean, we just have to take it as we go, I mean everyone has to go through whatever, and it is not really a big thing, you know" (Crystal, 68 years).

> "I guess we have to accept these things. It is part of the ageing process and illness is something that happens as you get older" (Freya, 69 years).

In general, the interviews revealed an acceptance by older men and women of their life situation and an expectation that ill-health usually accompanies the process of ageing. The interviews suggest that they have also learnt to manage their chronic illnesses and they have moved on with their lives. Butler and Ciarrochi (2007) state that some older people appear to respond to problems of ageing and the impacts of these on their quality of life better than others (Butler & Ciarrochi, 2007). As people age, they may struggle with certain changes such as the reduced ability to participate in activities they feel are meaningful. However, coming to terms with these changes and accepting them as a part of the process of ageing may help maintain their quality of life and mental health when challenges emerge (Butler & Ciarrochi, 2007).

Older people also experienced economic hardships that imposed additional limitations on them. Most (16) participants relied only on old-age pensions as their main source of income. Four participants earned an extra income from working in addition to their old-age grant. In addition, the participants revealed that they were provided with some financial support from their adult children. A few reported that their children even paid for their medical insurance which took some of the burden off them. However, their medical insurance did not cover all their costs, thus requiring out-of-pocket expenditure. This is problematic as the main source of income for older people (at the time of the study) was the old-age grant of R1750, which was reported to not be adequate to cater for all of their needs. Moana was one of the participants who received the old grant but could not afford to pay for her medical insurance. However, it was covered by her children. She remarked positively: "*I am advantaged in that way because of the medical aid, which I would never be able to pay if it was not for my children. Because the medical aid is more than my pension*". Older people are grateful for receiving the old-age pension, but they are also aware that it does not cover their private healthcare. What is clear, however, is that they lean on others for support particularly other family members.

Choice of Health Services

Almost half the participants stated that they received their healthcare at public facilities, and the other half stated that they visited private facilities for their health conditions. These facilities included clinics, hospitals, and general practitioner surgeries. The most common reason for receiving assistance at government-provided facilities was affordability. Isabelle and Derrick stated that they went to government-provided health facilities as they were more affordable than private health facilities.

> "At the moment what I am doing, ever since my husband passed away, money is a bit tight, so what I do is go to the public clinic here, Redhill clinic. I take all my medication there" (Isabelle, 72 years).

"I do not have medical aid. I go to state run hospitals. The medication at the private hospital is so expensive and at the state hospital you get the same medication for actually next to nothing" (Derrick, 60 years).

Cyril and Gretel utilise public services because they are unable to afford private services. However, they felt that if they had the option, they would go to a private health facility. The perception of better quality private services was given as the main reason for the choice of private services.

"Government facility. There is no other option, and that is the most affordable option. Medical aid is unaffordable, I would like to have one. It would make life much easier" (Cyril, 63 years).

"I go to the government. I never actually chose to. I am forced to because I am financially not well off and just with the pension money, I have to do it. I do not have medical aid, I cannot afford it" (Gretel, 62 years).

Obara also stated that she would prefer private healthcare as she receives poor service from the government-provided facility where they are constantly losing her paperwork and are unhelpful in solving her health problems.

"I would prefer to go private. In the [government-provided] hospital they are forever losing my chart. Then, at the same time I have to go do a lot of running around—upstairs, downstairs, and stuff like that, for them to find my chart. And they do not look for it, they send you to look for it. I finish off so late, and I am not at the age where I am going to take my time and the whole day before I come home. We go there and we need to come home quickly and rest" (Obara, 64 years).

Jessie stated that while she had no medical aid, she preferred to visit her private general practitioner for her healthcare as it was convenient for her to travel back and forth from the facility because it was not far from her residence. She is able to walk to and from the doctor. She managed her doctor's fees with the money from her pension, and when she goes for blood tests, her daughters help to finance some of the costs.

> "Just the private general practitioner doctor, because it is closer to home and I can just take a walk, it is not far from home. No medical aid, because we are not working at the moment, it is just me and my husband, we are living on a pension. If I go for blood tests, my daughters pay for me. It would have been nice; it would have made things easier for me" (Jessie, 60 years).

There is a huge divide in the quality of health services offered by the different sectors. It is clear that most of the older Indians would prefer to visit private health facilities and, sometimes, they are also prepared to pay for these services even if they cannot afford them. Another study found that older patients use commercial health providers because of the unavailability, poor quality, or age insensitivity of services at government-provided health facilities (Aboderin & Beard, 2015). Although economic factors are significant, there are other factors which influence people's choice of service including access to medical aid, and attitudes to and perceptions about particular services.

Moana explained that even though she visits a private healthcare facility and has a medical aid, all of her treatment is not covered by the plan which only covers the cost of her chronic medication. Nisha expressed the same.

> "Because I pay the hospital plan, chronic medication is covered to a certain extent by the hospital plan. But all my medication for anything extra, for my bone pain or hot flushes and all that, vitamin C, vitamin D, that is all absolutely necessary for my wellbeing, I have got to buy with my own money" (Moana, 68 years).

> "I go to private hospital because of medical aid. It does cover expenses but certain things I have to pay for" (Nisha, 78 years).

A number of participants are unable to afford medical aid, and they depended on their children to fund their medical costs. Elena is able to receive healthcare at a private hospital as her daughter pays for the medical aid for her, highlighting the importance of family support for older people. She recognises her fortunate situation and is grateful for the support she gets from her daughter.

> "I go to private hospital because I am on a medical aid, and my daughter pays for me" (Elena, 80 years).

However, not all older people were satisfied with private health services. For most of the participants, costs are a major concern. Freya has a medical aid and visits a private health provider, but she stated that she was not satisfied with her healthcare. This was due to her concerns about the high costs of private healthcare.

> "This healthcare that I have at the moment is quite expensive and sometimes it can have an impact on my savings, so if there is something that will provide a similar healthcare which is cheaper, that will definitely benefit me" (Freya, 69 years).

Despite efforts to redress the inherent inequalities of apartheid, there are some glaring disparities within the healthcare system between the private and public health sectors (Maphumulo & Bhengu, 2019). These inequalities were also evident in the study with half of the older Indian adults stating that they received their healthcare at government-provided healthcare facilities as they were free or affordable, whilst the other half did so in the private sector. The public health sector is under a lot of pressure due to the fact that most people cannot afford private-sector health services, and only around 17% of the population have access to a medical aid (Statistics South Africa, 2019).

A study by Kon and Lackan (2008) found that even though South Africa's health system has stark inadequacies, public perceptions of how the government is conducting healthcare service provision are not entirely negative, as the majority of Black Africans and Coloureds believed that the government was adequately improving healthcare services whilst the opposite was found for Whites and Indians. However, this study is relatively outdated, and no new data has been published, which is problematic as social issues such as inequality are increasing rapidly. There is the perception that private healthcare provides a better quality service. Other reasons suggested for the use of costly private healthcare treatment is that it is likely to be timely and more efficient.

Barriers to Access

Both men and women identified many barriers to accessing services, ranging from physical to functional, and economic factors. Most health facilities are located in areas which are difficult to access easily, especially for frail older people. While a few participants who were in better health managed to drive themselves to their health facility, most had to secure private transportation to get to the nearest health facility. Most often, they were driven to health facilities by family members, usually their children. This was the most relied-on transportation method for the participants, once again highlighting the importance of family support for older people.

Some participants rely on public transportation to reach health services, which is very challenging for them. Participants reported that public transport is not user friendly for older people, and they also have to walk a long distance before they get transportation, because it does not come close to their place of residence. Even if public transportation is available, travelling alone is also problematic. They complained that public transport is often not reliable, and as a result, they get to the health facility late.

> "Sometimes I have a problem because I am let down by my transport, and go late to the hospital" (Katherine, 64 years).

> "I have to leave home very early, and transport is a problem. We do not have buses near my house so we have to walk a long distance to take the taxi, and long distance to get back home. For hospital, I have to go early to follow the queues. If you do not go early, you have to wait even longer and may not get your medication" (Gretel, 62 years).

The physical conditions of older people also make it difficult for them to access health services. Anna and Obara expressed that their body pains often prevent them from going to health facilities. Obara observed "*sometimes I have problems with my legs, so I find it hard to go*". At health facilities, clients have to spend long hours in queues. Participants complained that the waiting time for the consultation was unreasonably long. Long waiting times have been shown to be an important reason for the relatively high rates of programme- and method-discontinuation and may sometimes serve to discourage potential clients from seeking services, as shown by Huntington and Schuler (1993). Anna observed that she developed "*back pains while waiting to be seen by a health provider*".

One of the recurring issues in the study was that the medical aid did not cover the cost of all treatment, and as a result, they have to pay the excess themselves. This is problematic as they are often unemployed and rely on the state pension that is often not adequate to meet their needs, or they have to rely on their families for financial support. It was often reported by older men and women that medical insurance did not cover all the medical expenses of the participants. The medical aid does not cover all the costs, requiring out-of-pocket expenditure. This is explained by Nisha: "*My medical aid only pays for some of my tablets. What they do not pay for, I use my pension for that*". Osman (2019) explains that medical aid savings are mainly used for acute expenditures, such as general doctor visits, and chronic medication is not always paid for as it would run the risk of depleting their medical savings. Self-payment gaps occur when the medical aid account becomes depleted over time. Some participants stated that they need financial assistance because their medical aid does not cover all their medical expenses, resulting in them having to use their pension for the extra medication.

Anthony and Isabelle described the challenges they experience in meeting their health needs. Anthony experienced trouble with his medical aid while Isabelle struggled to meet health needs with just the government pension.

> "One of my medical aids had paid for the doctor (general practitioner) but refused to pay for the hospital, so I had to immediately change that to another medical aid, which then paid for hospital, but not the doctor" (Anthony, 72 years).

> "Sometimes you know if you collect your grant and you really want to buy like tablets or something, you cannot afford it and then you have to wait another month. I do not worry the children to help me" (Isabelle, 72 years).

The older men and women stated that there are often times where the hospital fails to provide all the required medication to them, leaving them with no choice but to buy them. Obara, Cyril, and Jessie explain that they are unable to meet some of their healthcare needs due to not being able to afford them.

> "Sometimes I do need certain medications the hospital does not give, so I find it hard. I have to make do without it because I cannot afford it" (Obara, 64 years).

> "Yes, maybe traction or something for my back because I have got sciatica in the leg nerve so sometimes to wake up from the bed and to even walk becomes a problem. And back traction costs a lot" (Cyril, 63 years).

> "Well, you have to stick to a certain diet because of diabetes, and diet food is a bit expensive, so if it was cheaper, it would have been nice. I just have to make do with what is affordable and sometimes what is affordable may not be good for the health" (Jessie, 60 years).

The lack of reliable transport was also a barrier to accessing healthcare. It was reported that public transport was not age-friendly nor was it accessible as they still had to walk some distance to get public transport. This also results in late arrivals at healthcare facilities, missed appointments, and delayed treatment. Without transport, it is very difficult for older people to travel to health facilities especially those with disabilities and frailties and other elements that prevent them from walking long distances (Aboyade et al., 2016; Vergunst et al., 2015). Missed appointments with doctors or delayed treatment negatively affects the consistency in the management of non-communicable diseases (Syed et al., 2013) which are already poorly managed in Africa (Aboyade et al., 2016). Without the support of family, many older men and women would not be able to access vital healthcare.

The Importance of Family

Families, in particular, play a very instrumental role in the lives of older people. This is probably a coping mechanism that older people use to move on instead of being hampered by chronic illness. In the Indian community, there is a strong emphasis on family cohesion and traditions which may also be linked to the prominent religious importance of the family unit, especially among Hindus. Family systems were often strengthened by the fact that the younger generation lived with the older generation under the same family roof, especially young males and their spouses. This reinforces the notion that younger members of the family would often take care of older members as they grow older.

It was not uncommon for the majority of older people to state that their children pay for their medical insurance or that they provide them with transportation to receive healthcare. This accentuates the significance of family support for older people and the close-knit family structure of Indians. In traditional Indian societies, older people were primarily taken care of by their families, mainly their children. Traditional norms and culture among the Indian population have been passed down for generations. These norms place high value on older people, and thus, they are respected because of their age (Sinha, 1984). Indians, being family-orientated and promoting familial collectivism and cohesion, are also heavily involved in caring for family members and are important support structures for older people (Chadda & Deb, 2013). This traditional social institution has been endured through ages and influences the lives of the individuals within it. The experiences of older people in the Indian community of Avoca may be somewhat different to that of the larger South African older persons community; this study highlighted the reliance on familial networks in meeting the healthcare needs of older people.

In sub-Saharan Africa, family is one of the main sources of support for older people (Nzima & Maharaj, 2020). This is also true for many other traditional societies, such as those in India, China, and South Africa, especially in areas where there is a lack of nursing homes or other facilities that are required to treat older people as they become more frail (Ren & Treiman, 2015; Schatz et al., 2015). However, this is threatened due to changing societal norms which alter cultures and change family structures (Panigrahi, 2013). These traditions and norms are increasingly eroded by a number of factors including urbanisation and migration of children. This is also disconcerting as it was found that Indians in South Africa had a higher annual growth rate among older people aged 60 and older when compared to other groups. The median age for Indians increased more than all the other population groups between 1996 and 2001, suggesting a higher ageing rate within this group (Statistics South Africa, 2014). In addition, between 2001 and 2011, the dependency ratio between older people and working-age adult Indians also increased, indicating and highlighting that a greater amount of family support and care is required for older people (Statistics South Africa, 2014).

Conclusion

Living in poor health is a daily reality for older people. Chronic illness and multi-morbidities are increasingly common at older ages, especially among Indians in South Africa. These health conditions create an increased demand for health services, which older people access at both public and private health facilities. However, a greater dependence on health services is not without both financial and institutional barriers. In the absence of family support, many older Indian men and women would not have access to healthcare. Finance has a major influence on overcoming these barriers as most of the reasons for the use of particular health services boil down to affordability and accessibility. Policies and programmes that aim to assist older people, such as social grants and cash transfer programmes, may assist with improving access to health services. This will in turn assist with poverty reduction by improving quality of life, thereby increasing productivity and preserving livelihoods (Gresh & Maharaj, 2013). Health services for older people must be safe, effective, efficient, and responsive without imposing fiscal burdens on individuals and their families, and this is instrumental in the achievement of the goal of universal healthcare coverage (Suzman et al., 2015). Even though traditional Indian culture and norms prescribe family-based care, the magnitude of the healthcare needs of older people in sub-Saharan Africa can no longer be catered for by family alone. Therefore, there is a need for interventions that amalgamate family-based care with formal support systems (Adamek et al., 2020).

Acknowledgements This chapter is based on a Masters dissertation by Sachin Sewpersad, under the supervision of Pranitha Maharaj, at the University of KwaZulu-Natal.

References

Aboderin, I. A., & Beard, J. R. (2015). Older people's health in sub-Saharan Africa. *The Lancet, 385*(9968), 9–11.

Aboyade, O. M., Beauclair, R., Mbamalu, O. N., Puoane, T. R., & Hughes, G. D. (2016). Health-seeking behaviours of older black women living with non-communicable diseases in an urban township in South Africa. *BMC Complementary and Alternative Medicine, 16*(1), 1–9.

Adamek, M. E., Chane, S., & Kotecho, M. G. (2020). Family and kin care of elders in sub-Saharan Africa. In P. Maharaj (Ed.), *Health and care in old age in Africa*. Routledge.

Adhikari, D., & Rijal, D. P. (2014). Factors Affecting Health Seeking Behavior of Senior Citizens of Dharan. *Journal of Nobel Medical College, 4*(1), 57–63.

Ameh, S., Gomez-Olive, F. X., Kahn, K., Tollman, S. M., & Klipstein-Grobusch, K. (2014). Predictors of healthcare use by adults 50 years and over in a rural South African setting. *Global Health Action, 7*(1), 25087686.

Bähler, C., Huber, C. A., Brüngger, B., & Reich, O. (2015). Multimorbidity, healthcare utilization and costs in an elderly community-dwelling population: A claims data based observational study. *BMC Health Services Research, 15*(1), 1–12.

Bigala, P., & Ayiga, N. (2014). Prevalence and predictors of elder abuse in Mafikeng Local Municipality in South Africa. *African Population Studies, 28*(1), 463–474.

Butler, J., & Ciarrochi, J. (2007). Psychological acceptance and quality of life in the elderly. *Quality of Life Research, 16*(4), 607–615.

Chadda, R. K., & Deb, K. S. (2013). Indian family systems, collectivistic society and psychotherapy. *Indian Journal of Psychiatry, 55*(2), 299.

Chassin, M. R., & Loeb, J. M. (2013). High-reliability healthcare: Getting there from here. *The Milbank Quarterly, 91*(3), 459–490.

Dokpesi, A. (2017). Senior Citizens Health Insurance Programme (SCHIP): A policy framework for healthy ageing in Nigeria. *Ageing International, 42*, 290–305.

Gresh, A., & Maharaj, P. (2013). Policy and programme responses. In P. Maharaj (Ed.), *Aging and health in Africa*. Springer.

Hasumi, T., & Jacobsen, K. H. (2014). Healthcare service problems reported in a national survey of South Africans. *International Journal for Quality in Healthcare, 26*(4), 482–489.

Huntington, D., & Schuler, S. R. (1993). The simulated client method: Evaluating client-provider interactions in family planning clinics. *Studies in Family Planning, 24*(3), 187–193.

Kelly, G., Mrengqwa, L., & Geffen, L. (2019). "They don't care about us": Older people's experiences of primary healthcare in Cape Town, South Africa. *BioMedical Central Geriatrics, 19*(1), 1–14.

Kon, Z. R., & Lackan, N. (2008). Ethnic disparities in access to care in post-apartheid South Africa. *American Journal of Public Health, 98*(12), 2272–2277.

Liu, Y.-B., Liu, L., Li, Y.-F., & Chen, Y.-L. (2015). Relationship between health literacy, health-related behaviors and health status: A survey of elderly Chinese. *International Journal of Environmental Research and Public Health, 12*(8), 9714–9725.

Maharaj, P. (2013). Introduction. In P. Maharaj (Ed.), *Aging and health in Africa*. Springer.

Maharaj, P., & Cleland, J. (2005). Integration of sexual and reproductive health services in KwaZulu-Natal, South Africa. *Health Policy and Planning, 20*(5), 310–318.

Maphumulo, W. T., & Bhengu, B. R. (2019). Challenges of quality improvement in the healthcare of South Africa post-apartheid: A critical review. *Curationis, 42*(1), 1–9.

Mtapuri, O., & Tinarwo, P. (2021). From apartheid to democracy: Patterns and trends of inequality in South Africa. *Southern African Journal of Demography, 21*(1), 104.

Nzima, D., & Maharaj, P. (2020). Long-term care for the elderly in sub-Saharan Africa. In P. Maharaj (Ed.), *Health and care in old age in Africa*. Routledge.

Osman, L. (2019). Why doesn't my medical aid pay for it? *SA Pharmacist's Assistant, 19*(1), 2–4.

Panigrahi, A. K. (2013). Living arrangements of elderly in India: A comparative study of Uttar Pradesh and Kerala. *Indian Journal of Gerontology, 27*(3), 495.

Prabhakaran, D., Jeemon, P., & Roy, A. (2016). Cardiovascular diseases in India: Current epidemiology and future directions. *Circulation, 133*(16), 1605–1620.

Prakaschandra, D. R., Esterhuizen, T. M., Motala, A. A., Gathiram, P., & Naidoo, D. P. (2016). High prevalence of cardiovascular risk factors in Durban South African Indians: The Phoenix lifestyle project. *South African Medical Journal, 106*(3), 284–289.

Ralston, M., Schatz, E., Menken, J., Gómez-Olivé, F. X., & Tollman, S. (2016). Who benefits—Or does not—From South Africa's old age pension? Evidence from characteristics of rural pensioners and non-pensioners. *International Journal of Environmental Research and Public Health, 13*(1), 85.

Ren, Q., & Treiman, D. J. (2015). Living arrangements of the elderly in China and consequences for their emotional well-being. *Chinese Sociological Review, 47*(3), 255–286.

Schatz, E., Madhavan, S., Collinson, M., Gómez-Olivé, F. X., & Ralston, M. (2015). Dependent or productive? A new approach to understanding the social positioning of older South Africans through living arrangements. *Research on Aging, 37*(6), 581–605.

Schoeman, T. (2018). The spatial influence of apartheid on the South African city. *The Geography Teacher, 15*(1), 29–32.

Seekings, J. (2008). The continuing salience of race: Discrimination and diversity in South Africa. *Journal of Contemporary African Studies, 26*(1), 1–25.

Sekhejane, P. R. (2013). *South African National Health Insurance (NHI) policy: Prospects and challenges for its efficient implementation.* Africa Institute of South Africa.

Sinha, D. (1984). Some recent changes in the Indian family and their implications for socialization. *Indian Journal of Social Work, 45*(3), 271–286.

Statistics South Africa. (2014). *Census 2011: Profile of older persons in South Africa.* Statistics South Africa.

Statistics South Africa. (2019). *Vulnerable groups indicator report 2017.* Statistics South Africa.

Statistics South Africa. (2021). *Mid-year population estimates 2021.* Statistics South Africa.

Statistics South Africa. (2022). *Mid-year population estimates 2022.* Statistics South Africa.

Streatfield, P. K., Khan, W. A., Bhuiya, A., Alam, N., Sié, A., Soura, A. B., Bonfoh, B., Ngoran, E. K., Weldearegawi, B., Jasseh, M., & Oduro, A. (2014). Cause-specific mortality in Africa and Asia: Evidence from INDEPTH health and demographic surveillance system sites. *Global Health Action, 7*(1), 25377324.

Suzman, R., Beard, J. R., Boerma, T., & Chatterji, S. (2015). Health in an ageing world—What do we know? *The Lancet, 385*(9967), 484–486.

Syed, S. T., Gerber, B. S., & Sharp, L. K. (2013). Traveling towards disease: Transportation barriers to healthcare access. *Journal of Community Health, 38*(5), 976–993.

Troeger, C., Blacker, B., Khalil, I. A., Rao, P. C., Cao, J., Zimsen, S. R., Albertson, S. B., Deshpande, A., Farag, T., Abebe, Z., & Adetifa, I. M. O. (2018). Estimates of the global, regional, and national morbidity, mortality, and aetiologies of lower respiratory infections in 195 countries, 1990–2016: A systematic analysis for the Global Burden of Disease Study 2016. *The Lancet Infectious Diseases, 18*(11), 1191–1210.

Vergunst, R., Swartz, L., Mji, G., MacLachlan, M., & Mannan, H. (2015). 'You must carry your wheelchair'–barriers to accessing healthcare in a South African rural area. *Global Health Action, 8*(1), 29003.

Wandera, S. O., Kwagala, B., & Ntozi, J. (2015). Prevalence and risk factors for self-reported non-communicable diseases among older Ugandans: A cross-sectional study. *Global Health Action, 8*(1), 27923.

World Health Organization (WHO). (2020). *Guidance on COVID-19 for the care of older people and people living in long-term care facilities, other non-acute care facilities and home care*. World Health Organization.

Zeh, P., Sandhu, H., Cannaby, A. M., & Sturt, J. (2014). Cultural barriers impeding ethnic minority groups from accessing effective diabetes care services: A systematic review of observational studies. *Divers Equal Healthcare, 11*(1), 9–33.

Zhou, F., Yu, T., Du, R., Fan, G., Liu, Y., Liu, Z., Xiang, J., Wang, Y., Song, B., Gu, X., & Guan, L. (2020). Clinical course and risk factors for mortality of adult inpatients with COVID-19 in Wuhan, China: A retrospective cohort study. *The Lancet, 395*(10229), 1054–1062.

8

Understanding Dementia and Elder Abuse in South Africa: The Challenge of 'Ageing in Place' with Dignity

Roxanne Jacobs, Nicolas Farina, and Marguerite Schneider

Abstract Dementia is often not recognised as a serious health condition in South Africa and goes undiagnosed or misdiagnosed, while the care falls primarily within an unprepared family. While South Africa's policy environment supports the philosophy of 'ageing in place' or 'active ageing', the country faces many challenges that threaten ageing in place with dignity where older persons are valued, respected, and treated ethically. This chapter describes the realities of people with dementia and their families in South Africa and shows how unsupported environments threaten the achievement of 'ageing in place' with dignity. The chapter provides an understanding of dementia in context and shows how

---

R. Jacobs (✉) • M. Schneider
Alan J. Flisher Centre for Public Mental Health, Department of Psychiatry and Mental Health, University of Cape Town, Cape Town, South Africa
e-mail: roxanne.jacobs@uct.ac.za; marguerite.schneider@uct.ac.za

N. Farina
Community and Primary Care Research Group, University of Plymouth, Plymouth, UK
e-mail: nicolas.farina@plymouth.ac.uk

P. Maharaj (ed.), *Navigating Ageing in South Africa*, Sustainable Development Goals Series, https://doi.org/10.1007/978-981-97-9088-3_8

unsupported needs lead to self-isolation and risk of elder abuse. For most South Africans, ageing is hard and an undignified experience. Dignified ageing requires support that includes public education and training, adequate service development, and strengthening culturally acceptable support for older persons and their families.

Keywords Elder abuse • Dementia • Ageing-in-place • South Africa

Introduction

Dementia is currently not recognised as a serious health condition in South Africa and is largely accepted by communities and some health and social care professionals as a 'normal part of ageing'. In South Africa, dementia often goes undiagnosed, whilst care and support fall to the family. Individuals with dementia and their families in South Africa encounter significant levels of stigma, which manifest as structural, internalised, and negative public beliefs (Jacobs et al., 2022b). Consequently, these adverse beliefs and responses often delay help-seeking and contribute to self-isolation, as families actively shield their loved ones with dementia from potentially harmful reactions beyond their immediate circle. The health and social care needs of people with dementia often go unmet, with families shouldering the responsibility of care largely unsupported by any formal care services that educate, empower, and support family carers to adequately respond to their needs.

South Africa's policy environment supports the philosophy of 'ageing in place' or 'active ageing' where the protection and inclusion of older persons in daily living and decision-making at home and within their communities are promoted (Jordan, 2009; WHO, 2002). While this philosophy is commendable, the country faces many challenges that threaten 'ageing in place' with dignity where older persons are valued, respected, and treated ethically. Crime and violence in South Africa are documented as one of the highest in the world—that is six times higher than the global average (Peden et al., 2002), with very little known and published about violence, crime, and abuse against older persons in this context. Even less is known about older persons living with dementia and their vulnerability to violence, abuse, and exploitation. People with dementia often require assisted self-care and support as the condition progresses, with later stages increasingly affecting the individual's functioning, communication, and self-care (Downes et al., 2013; WHO, 2019). Globally, these realities of caregiving for someone with dementia have been linked to a greater risk of elder abuse and neglect (Campbell-Reay & Browne, 2001; Downes et al., 2013).

This chapter describes the realities of people with dementia and their families in South Africa and shows how living with dementia in an unsupported context threatens the achievement of 'ageing in place' with dignity. It provides an understanding of dementia in context and shows how unsupported needs of people living with dementia and their families pose risks for self-isolation and elder abuse.

Understanding Dementia and the Risk of Elder Abuse

Globally, 50 million people are estimated to be living with dementia, and this is expected to increase to 152.8 million by 2050 (Nichols et al., 2022). Dementia prevalence is, however, less established for African contexts. Limited data available on dementia in Africa estimated the four Sub-Saharan regions to range between 2% and 4% (Prince et al., 2013). Dementia prevalence for South Africa has also not been established conclusively. Aside from one localised study conducted in the Eastern Cape (De Jager et al., 2017), the STRIDE (Strengthening Responses to Dementia in Developing Countries) project was the only attempt to identify dementia at the community level across two provinces, Limpopo and the Western Cape, using the 10/66 short algorithm for diagnosing probable dementia amongst people 65 years and older (for more information see Farina et al., 2023). This study estimated dementia at 12.5% in South Africa, with only 0.5% of older persons having received an actual diagnosis (Farina et al., 2023).

Dementia is an umbrella term that describes a group of neurodegenerative diseases that are progressive and symptomatic of memory decline, decreased mental ability and loss of executive functioning that is severe enough to impede daily functioning (Alzheimer's Association, 2019; WHO, 2019). Symptoms vary from person to person and inevitably progresses over time, becoming more pronounced as it starts affecting the individual's behaviour (Downes et al., 2013). For example, confusion and noticeable mood disturbances, such as increased aggression and agitation, are usually uncharacteristic of their personality before dementia. At later stages of dementia, the person has increased difficulty recognising family and friends, and progressively requires assisted self-care and support (Downes et al., 2013; WHO, 2019).

Caring for someone living with dementia is physically, emotionally, and financially demanding. It involves providing assisted self-care to the ageing family member, managing challenging behavioural symptoms, making medical decisions, and providing support for end-of-life care. Dementia often exceeds the care demands of other chronic conditions (Prince et al., 2015) and is especially taxing when struggling to cope with unmanaged symptoms due to a lack of diagnosis and health and social care responses and support. Unsurprisingly, carers of people with dementia are at increased risk of poor health outcomes themselves and are known to struggle with anxiety and depression, maladaptive coping (e.g. confrontative and avoidance strategies), and caregiver burden (Cooper et al., 2007).

While the risk of negative health outcomes for unsupported carers is universal, younger carers are more likely to struggle with anxiety when caring for a dementia care-recipient with unmanaged behavioural symptoms (Cooper et al., 2007). Irrespective of carer age, aggressive symptoms from care-recipients are globally found to act as triggers of reciprocal violence in care dyads (Baharudin et al., 2019; Downes et al., 2013). Unsupported family carers are therefore vulnerable to an increased risk of abusing and, in certain circumstances, feel victimised themselves. In South Africa, there are many challenges that provide unsupported environments for people with dementia and their families. A context of widespread poverty, stigma, and a lack of dementia awareness, limited or no access to diagnosis and support, leaves families completely unprepared and ill-equipped to meet the care needs of someone with dementia. A major focus of this chapter is to unpack these realities and discuss the challenges that increase the risk to older persons, people with dementia and their families in South Africa.

The Privilege of a Dementia Diagnosis

Access to a dementia diagnosis, treatment, and care is privileged in South Africa, with great variation in the knowledge, skill, and training on dementia amongst healthcare professionals (Jacobs et al., 2022a; Kalula & Petros, 2011). Despite active redress by government to improve equal access to healthcare, public health services remain limited due to extended queuing systems, long waiting lists, and serious limitations in human, financial, and technological resources to support much-needed services for older people and their families (Mahlathi & Dlamini, 2015; South African Government, 2017). An estimated 79% of medical doctors in the country are located within the private sector, with only 16% of South Africans having access to medical insurance to financially support access to these services (Mahlathi & Dlamini, 2015; Rawat, 2012; Statistics South Africa, 2019).

Currently, there are no dementia-specific services at primary healthcare level in South Africa, with less than ten geriatricians and five geriatric psychiatrists to serve over 5.5 million older persons in the country (Kalula & Petros, 2011; Statistics South Africa, 2021). Whilst current healthcare policy does little to directly address the needs of people with dementia, existing inequalities in the healthcare system amplify the inadequacies in dementia responsiveness. As such, most people with dementia in South Africa are living without a diagnosis and without any formal treatment or care.

Access to a timely diagnosis is critical and allows access to information, resources, and support for the older person and their family. Non-pharmaceutical responses may extend and improve quality of life and allow people with dementia and their families to plan for the future (Alzheimer's Disease International, 2024). Whilst pharmacology interventions help manage symptoms for a limited time, new medications are coming to the market that may reduce underlying pathology for people with early Alzheimer's Disease (Van Van Dyck et al., 2023). However, without the necessary health and support services to respond to a diagnosis, living with dementia with dignity is challenging in South Africa. Pockets of care are available to those who can afford it, while the majority of South Africans rely on state-provided healthcare services that largely respond to competing health priorities such as early childhood development, HIV/AIDS, TB, and other non-communicable diseases. As populations age and live longer, dementia risk increases along with a growing need for care and support. Nurses are the backbone of primary healthcare in South Africa and the pillars of the country's public healthcare system. To date, geriatrics and dementia are not included in nurse's training curricula, and the knowledge and skill to respond to dementia is as unequal as access to diagnostic services. These structural barriers keep dementia hidden and families isolated as they navigate the realities of living with this condition.

Dementia Stigma: The Power of Awareness and Education

Stigma, dangerous beliefs, and misconceptions about dementia play a significant role in delaying help-seeking behaviour and placing older persons at risk of neglect, violence, abuse, and, in some cases, death. Across the world, various cultures and belief systems have responded differently to the symptoms of dementia (Alzheimer's Disease International, 2024). Countries such as Ghana (Ofori-Atta et al., 2010), Nigeria (Adewuya & Oguntade, 2007), Uganda (Quinn & Knifton, 2014), and Tanzania (Mushi et al., 2014) have reflected on how local cultural belief systems often brand older women who exhibit strange behaviours (often associated with dementia) as 'witches', making them targets for victimisation through public acts of violence and death (Benade, 2012; Khonje et al., 2015). Religions across the world may directly or indirectly facilitate these beliefs through their explanations for illness and strange behaviours (e.g. they are the result of 'evil spirits', 'possession', and 'punishment')

(Ally & Laher, 2008; Spitte et al., 2019). Stigma and fear of harmful community beliefs may lead someone with dementia and their families into hiding (Mkhonto & Hanssen, 2018). While more information on dementia stigma in South Africa is published elsewhere (see Jacobs et al., 2022b), experts by experience (i.e. people with dementia and their carers) have reported strategies that include (i) selective disclosing of diagnosis/symptoms only to the most trusted family members; (ii) masking vulnerability where a person with dementia publicly displays behaviours that project an image of well-being and being active to ward off suspicion; and (iii) self-isolation to prevent others from noticing symptoms. These effects of stigma and the fear of harmful beliefs therefore negatively influence help-seeking behaviour and their care.

In South Africa, stigma is also found at a structural level where institutionalised norms of dismissing dementia as a 'normal part of ageing' delay or prevent people with dementia from accessing diagnosis and care. Primary healthcare workers and service users alike report beliefs that 'nothing can be done' for someone with dementia, thus constraining opportunities for supportive responses. While lack of training and information about dementia at primary healthcare level is a reality, where knowledge does in fact exist, community healthcare workers may actually encourage the belief that dementia is a 'normal part of ageing' within communities to deliberately counter harmful beliefs that may place older persons (especially women) at risk of stigmatisation and harmful labelling associated with violent community reactions. Voicing of certain beliefs to shield people with dementia about the realities of living with dementia in South Africa can also be observed in the belief that 'nothing can be done'. The belief that 'nothing can be done' for someone with dementia may be perpetuated by a lack of available health, care, and support services where doctors can refer their patients to. These realities reflect a dementia-blind healthcare system where fragmented care pathways deny timeous access to diagnosis, care, and support. In turn, a dementia-blind system also perpetuates a lack of public knowledge and education about dementia as a serious health condition that is not a 'normal part of ageing'.

In the absence of supportive responses to dementia at both the community and structural levels, families often navigate the realities of caring for a family member with dementia in isolation. Primary healthcare systems can therefore play a direct role in challenging harmful community beliefs about dementia-related symptoms. Increasing access to diagnosis, education and understanding of the condition at community and macro-levels has the power to protect older persons (especially women) from abuse, and where relevant, violent community reactions that marginalise and restrict the movements of older Black women.

Factors Increasing the Risk of Abuse for Older Persons in South Africa

Poverty, Unemployment, and Substance Abuse

In South Africa, 9.2% of the population are 60 years and older (Statistics South Africa, 2021), and this is projected to increase to 15.4% in 2050 and 27.8% by 2100 (United Nations, 2015). In a context of widespread poverty, unemployment, and migrant labour practices, pensions often become the only stable income within a household. Widespread unemployment and the lack of financial resources for younger people therefore put pressure on pension incomes to support entire families, where adult children become dependent on the older person's pension and their labour to rear grandchildren. While remaining active members within a family support 'active ageing' and 'ageing in place' philosophies, the context of poverty and unemployment adds an enormous burden on older person's time, labour, and finances.

South Africans also experience very high rates of substance abuse where 10.3% of adults are estimated to consume alcohol and 8.6% consume illicit drugs at harmful levels (Pengpid et al., 2021). The presence of substance abuse in the family may be a trigger for elder abuse. If the older person is a source of income to the family, older adults may become the target for financial exploitation to support these family addictions. Substance abuse within the household is also strongly associated with violent behaviour, maladaptive coping, and mental health challenges such as depression and anxiety—all well-known risk factors for elder abuse (Downes et al., 2013).

Spirituality and Socio-Cultural Beliefs

Spirituality is an important feature of South African culture, though it would be reductionist to say that there is a single, unified culture. South Africa is a multi-cultural country with a myriad of beliefs, religions, and practices. Traditional healing falls within broader understandings of spirituality and is a socially acceptable practice amongst certain cultures in the country to identify and treat conditions believed to be unresponsive to biomedicine (Audet et al., 2017). Traditional ideologies are not universal or homogenous; however, a common belief is that the causes of some conditions, diseases or misfortunes are social in origin (Mkhonto & Hanssen, 2018). This is especially true for any conditions that relate to mental health, where traditional healers are often the first port of call for families seeking help, treatment, and care for an affected loved one. Traditional healers are believed to be able to identify and treat conditions caused by social misconduct, spirits, spells, and witchcraft whereas biomedicine is unable to diagnose and treat (Audet et al., 2017). They speak the local languages of the person seeking help, are often living within close proximity, are easily available for consultation, and are believed to spend more time explaining problems, causes, and treatments to patients. Therefore, traditional healers are often preferred over mainstream biomedical approaches or, in some cases, used in conjunction with biomedicine (Audet et al., 2017). It is estimated that 72% of South Africans consult traditional healers (Sobiecki, 2014).

While spirituality is an important source of support for many South Africans, certain socio-cultural beliefs have also been linked to a greater risk of violence and abuse against older persons. In South Africa, as well as other African countries, women (especially black African women) can become targets of allegations of 'witchcraft'. While this phenomenon is not universal, pockets of these belief systems in South Africa identify older women in particular as 'witches' that are blamed for misfortunes or natural disasters affecting communities (e.g. droughts, disease, social problems) (Kalula & Petros, 2011; Kotzé, 2018; Mkhonto & Hanssen, 2018). These allegations have been linked to extreme forms of violence against older women, where victims and their families are assaulted, burned, and violently killed. Older people are deprived of their belongings, food, and shelter and are victims of violent sexual crimes perpetrated by family and strangers alike (SAHRC, 2015). In the absence of national surveillance data on such forms of violence, qualitative reports from civil society and human rights watchdog organisations reveal that undiagnosed dementia may have played a direct role in community's reaction to perceived erratic behaviour (SAHRC, 2015; SAPRA, 2014).

Dementia has therefore also been linked to allegations of 'witchcraft', where symptoms that include confusion, memory loss, or strange behaviours (like mood swings and erratic behaviour) are understood as 'bewitched', 'cursed', 'possessed', or 'punished' (Khonje et al., 2015). The lack of understanding in communities of dementia as a serious health condition amplifies this risk and sends people living with dementia and their families (where these believes are prevalent) into hiding, and negatively affecting their help-seeking behaviour (Jacobs et al., 2022b).

Families as First Responders and at Risk

In South Africa, families are a critical resource of support and care for dementia and are generally the first responders to the needs of older family members in need of care and support. However, as described above, traditional family structures are under enormous pressure to navigate the realities of adequately caring for someone living with dementia in resource-constrained and dementia-blind care systems. Dementia often leads to isolation, and without respite and adequate support, families can become hostile environments that place older persons at risk of harm, neglect, violence, and abuse.

Like dementia, awareness and education are also needed in understanding and adequately responding to elder abuse. Globally, definitions of elder abuse vary across cultures, contexts, time, and place (Moon & Benton, 2000). Despite these variations, universally, elder abuse remains largely hidden with an estimated 4% of cases actually being reported (WHO, 2016). Not much is known about elder abuse in South Africa, with a dearth of research on older persons (including dementia and abuse) and no formal systems of monitoring, surveillance, and reporting nationally. The following section describes the complexities in understanding and detecting elder abuse in a context of dementia and shows how leveraging existing local resources can channel support to older persons and their families in culturally acceptable ways.

Complexities in Understanding and Detecting Elder Abuse

In South Africa, elder abuse is defined by the South African Older Persons Act (no. 13 of 2006) as "*...any conduct of lack of appropriate action, occurring within any relationship where there is an expectation of trust, which causes harm or distress or is likely to cause harm or distress to an older person*" (Government Gazette, 2006). In line with the World Health Organization, this definition refers to acts that are intentional or reflect neglect and includes broad types of abuse that are physical, emotional, sexual, or financial (WHO, 2018).

Defining and understanding elder abuse in context is complex. Variations in definitions across the world add to this complexity as to what constitutes abuse is informed by the norms and values of a particular place, context, and time (Momtaz et al., 2013; Moon & Benton, 2000). A key element of elder abuse is that it occurs within a relationship of trust (Downes et al., 2013; Goergen & Beaulieu, 2013; Jackson, 2016). Earlier definitions excluded perpetrators who were not related to the older person but later evolved to include strangers who deliberately build trust in order to deceive and exploit (Goergen & Beaulieu, 2013; Jackson, 2016). For example, in South Africa, strangers target older people because of their age, assume vulnerability, and deliberately build trust to convince older people to sign papers to purchase furniture, sign over their pension, or property, without informed consent or realising that they are losing these assets. While the contract signed may be legally binding, the manner in which access to assets is obtained is inherently exploitative and constitutes financial abuse. In the absence of accessible legal support for the majority of older persons who cannot afford expensive lawyers, these acts from both family and strangers alike go largely unchallenged. Economic motivations for incapacitation claims or 'witchcraft' allegations have also been noted where family members, for example, a grandson denied an older woman access to her assets or confiscate her property for personal gain (Kotzé, 2018). Research on these issues is limited with very little known about the risks and social abuses that older persons, especially women in South Africa, face.

These risks are amplified when an older person has dementia or any form of disability or functional impairment. Known risk factors for older persons being vulnerable to abuse include their functional dependence, physical and mental health, and cognitive impairment (Pillemer et al., 2016). Older persons with cognitive impairments such as dementia are therefore at increased risk of abuse as these conditions compromise their ability to recognise, respond, and disclose abuse (Downes et al., 2013).

Drivers of Under-Reporting in South Africa

Globally, elder abuse is complex and often considered a hidden problem with one in six persons aged 60 years and older estimated to have experienced some form of abuse (WHO, 2016, 2017). The risk of elder abuse increases with increased care needs, with two out of three people with dementia being estimated to have experienced some form of abuse (WHO, 2016, 2017). Older persons themselves may hide abuse for reasons that include fear of retaliation, feelings of shame, and helplessness, or concern for getting the abuser in trouble or losing their financial support especially if the abuser is their adult child (WHO, 2016). Research globally has also noted that older persons may not recognise their situation as an abusive one, while persons with cognitive impairment are at increased risk because the condition may limit their insight, recall ability or communication skills to disclose (Downes et al., 2013).

Globally, as is in South Africa, under-reporting is driven by various factors. Reluctance from families, communities, and professionals alike is motivated by three main factors: (1) awareness of rights and insight to recognise their situation as an abusive one; (2) feelings of shame, helplessness, and discomfort in talking about (or confronting) their abusive situation; and (3) not knowing what to do, whom to report to, or what to expect when reporting abuse (Jacobs et al., 2022a). The latter refers to the fear of consequences, including fear of retaliation, becoming homeless or destitute, or isolated from familiar people and surroundings. These fears are driven by realities of reporting elder abuse in South Africa, whereby the older person is sometimes removed from their homes and placed in a place of safety while the perpetrator's life continues uninterrupted, until the investigation is completed. While these decisions are justified by the immediate need to protect the older person from a dangerous environment, the action itself becomes unjust as the victim of abuse potentially suffers secondary trauma because of being removed from their homes, loved ones, and broader sources of social support that could be instrumental in the older person's recovery from an abusive relationship. These fears of statutory responses therefore contribute to underreporting and continue to mask elder abuse within communities.

Alternative sources of support or formal/informal social services that respond to family intervention needs are largely unavailable. There are currently no specific organisations or dedicated non-government organisations (NGOs) that specialise in the provision of support services for elder abuse. The state relies heavily on the NGO sector to provide social services, but these NGOs are severely underfunded and unable to cope with current demands. Existing health and social care systems are ill-equipped to detect or respond to elder abuse as there is currently no standard way of screening for abuse, or adequate training for doctors, nurses, social workers, and allied health professionals to identify and respond to elder abuse. This lack of capacity of services is a serious problem with both community and systemic roots and continues to mask the needs for protection of older people.

Understanding how elder abuse is manifested locally directly relates to its criminalisation and adequate responses that provide support and protection to older persons. Elder abuse in South Africa is criminalised as a punishable offense, with the South African Older Persons Act (no. 13 of 2006) providing policy support for the promotion of older person's safety and well-being (Government Gazette, 2006). However, there is no public health strategy (or funding model) in place to guide implementation of policies that directly address elder abuse (or dementia), or guide intersectoral collaboration efforts to protect the health and safety of older persons in South Africa. For example, responding to elder abuse is a shared responsibility that involves various sectors, including policing, community safety, health and social care, social development, and the legal and judicial system. If pathways that promote intersectoral collaboration are not clearly defined, funded and capacitated, responses to elder abuse (and dementia) will remain fragmented and continue to occur in isolated pockets of care for those who can afford it.

Elder Abuse in the Context of Dementia

Understanding elder abuse and adequate responses to the needs of older persons and their families is complex. Elder abuse in the context of dementia is even more complex because progressing care demands occur on a spectrum over time that includes risk as family roles and responsibilities change in unsupportive environments. Not all perpetrators of abuse are equal in culpability (Jackson, 2016). Caring for someone with dementia demonstrates these nuances in understanding the complexities of elder abuse, culpability, and the necessary responses to protect older persons in their journey of ageing with dignity.

Globally, known risk factors of elder abuse perpetration include carers having poor social support, high levels of care burden, depression and psychopathology, and substance abuse (Downes et al., 2013). These risks for perpetration are often exacerbated by social determinants of violence such as poverty, inequality, and widespread unemployment that strain families and their resources. The vignette (the story of Granny M) below demonstrates a real-life scenario of a typical dementia care pathway in South Africa, where despite variations across cultures and socio-economic background, responses to an older person with dementia largely take place within the home—largely unsupported by formal and informal services. This vignette demonstrates the complexity of understanding elder abuse in the context of dementia and shows how culpability of abuse ranges on a spectrum of deliberate intentional acts, to neglect.

Scenario: The Story of Granny M

Granny M lives with her husband, adult son, and his wife and two children in a working-class community. The older couple live in the extended quarters at the back of a two-bedroom house. Granny M comes from a very religious family and was always very active in her community, while maintaining her household and assisting her adult children in caring for her grandchildren while they are at work at the nearby textile factories. Granny M has not been able to do her usual daily activities, with a growing need for assistance from her husband to wash and dress herself. She is no longer able to maintain the household, do the shopping, and cook and clean for them like she used to. Her family is growing concerned with her memory problems and her odd behaviour, and what people in the community might think if she continues to wear inappropriate clothes or disrobe in public. Granny M's son believes she is 'acting out' and 'looking for attention' as a way of manipulating them to spend more time with her, while her husband and older siblings believe that her distress is caused by the jealousies of others and that she needs to consult a spiritual leader to ease her suffering. This situation is causing distress and conflict within the family as these generations struggle to agree on how to respond to the care of Granny M.

As symptoms progress and become more noticeable, the immediate response of the family is to hide Granny M from social events and community activities, including preventing her from attending her religious meetings she used to frequent for fear that someone would notice changes in her behaviour and stigmatise the family. Immediate family members may downplay the severity of her symptoms and excuse her absence from broader social events being due to age-related health issues. Her family becomes more isolated and divided in making decisions about her care. Granny M is also receiving medical treatment for other conditions like hypertension and is accompanied by her son for check-ups for these pre-existing conditions. Seeking help for her hypertension act as a doorway for her son to consult the public health clinic staff on his concerns about his mother's odd behaviour and memory problems. Clinic staff identifies his concerns as a being a 'normal part of ageing', with no immediate treatment response. Later, she is misdiagnosed with depression and taking State-issued medications to respond to depressive symptoms. The effects of the misdiagnosis and incorrect medication worsen her symptoms and result in her husband secretly taking her to consult a spiritual healer, who prescribes traditional remedies to ease her suffering. Granny M is consuming remedies from both biomedical and traditional practices, with ingredients from both prescriptions worsening her condition. Her behavioural symptoms become unmanageable and are characterised by fluctuations between low mood and extreme lethargy and heightened displays of aggression.

(*continued*)

(continued)

Care for Granny M is unlikely to come from paid care arrangements and is absorbed within the family where eventually the daughter-in-law quits her job to care for her mother-in-law. This loss of income adds additional financial pressure on the family, with growing children and two ailing grandparents to care for and financially support. Unmanaged symptoms become increasingly difficult for the daughter-in-law to manage, despite the help of Granny M's husband when he's able to assist. Lately, he is unable to cope with the physical demands of his wife's care, as he struggles with his own health and finds it hard to deal with his wife's memory loss and difficult behaviour. The family feels alone and completely unprepared on how to deal with Granny M's behaviour. Her family is frustrated by her behaviour, and with mounting pressures to care for her, get her dressed, eat and attend to her hygiene, Granny M's husband and daughter-in-law find themselves having to be rough with her to get things done so that they can focus on other chores, childcare needs and urgent household responsibilities.

Granny M's condition progresses without formal support from any primary healthcare or community-based services. Her condition deteriorates rapidly as she loses her ability to speak, eat and other functional abilities. Granny M is likely to remain at home in the care of her family until the end of life.

The power of diagnosis and understanding dementia plays a crucial role in promoting active ageing and ageing with dignity in South Africa. While this scenario may vary across cultures and socio-economic backgrounds, a common thread remains that people with dementia in South Africa are likely to go undiagnosed or misdiagnosed, with families being completely unprepared and ill-equipped to adequately respond to care needs. For example, symptoms are often worsened by inadequate and/or inappropriate responses in both biomedical and traditional practices, rendering families unable to manage neuropsychiatric symptomatology, especially aggressive behaviours. Aggressive behaviours are known risk factors for elder abuse in dementia care scenarios and often trigger reciprocal violence from carers to cope with care demands (Downes et al., 2013) as a way to 'get things done'. Carers themselves feel victimised, and the increase in carer burden that results from unmanaged symptoms increases the risk of abuse and neglect, especially when maladaptive strategies are employed like avoidance (e.g. avoiding hygiene routines to avoid conflict and aggression) and substance use (e.g. coping with stress through harmful use of alcohol). Furthermore, for Granny M, as dementia progressed, she gradually lost her ability to communicate and was unable to indicate, for example, when and where she was experiencing pain. Not understanding how communication changes throughout the progression of the disease undermines the family's ability to detect and adequately respond to pain. These examples therefore show how neglect on the one hand can become a survival strategy to avoid conflict, and on the other hand, where family simply do not know what to look out for when caring for their family member with dementia. While this scenario is an oversimplification of the reality of dementia care within an unprepared and unsupported family, it does show the complexity in understanding what constitutes elder abuse and how culpability ranges from premeditated acts of abuse, to genuinely not knowing how to care for someone with dementia.

Recommendations for Strengthening Responses to Dementia and Elder Abuse

This chapter describes the realities of people with dementia in South Africa. It has shown how understanding dementia and elder abuse is complex and how various factors drive the under-reporting of abuse at family, community, and structural levels. Stigma and fear of harmful beliefs send families into hiding and delay help-seeking behaviours, while lack of awareness of dementia at both community and primary healthcare levels can leave families equally vulnerable in providing the needed care. Currently, South Africa has a long way to go to strengthen responses to dementia that will allow equal access to care, treatment, and the promotion of active ageing and ageing with dignity. However, despite these challenges, there are various strengths that a coordinated response to dementia can activate immediately to provide support to people with dementia and their families, including public education and training, improved services, supporting families, and bringing together traditional healing and biomedical approaches.

Public Education and Training

Public education and training are important first steps to combat stigma and harmful beliefs that negatively affect help-seeking behaviour and responses to care and support. Formalising basic dementia training within existing healthcare curricula for nurses, doctors, and allied health professionals, including community health workers, should be mandatory and part of standard care (currently, geriatrics is an elective).

Service Development for Dementia and Elder Abuse

Dementia can be integrated into public health strategies that historically have prioritised the health and well-being of the population, for example, the National Health Promotion Policy and Strategy (2014), the National Health Act (2003), and the Older Person's Act (2026). In the absence of a National Dementia Plan, these policies can be strengthened to guide and mandate coordinated responses that foster intersectoral collaboration to support the needs of those living with dementia, acknowledging the importance of families within our context. Currently, the South African policy environment locates the responsibility of care for older persons within the family without the necessary support in place to provide information, education, respite, and community-based care. While the promotion of keeping older persons active within their communities for as long as possible is commendable, the widespread lack of available support services creates vulnerabilities for abuse and neglect. Furthermore, responses to elder abuse should be linked to available home-based, community care and/or judicial services where needed—supported with a budget for programmes and services that are needed to promote prevention, disclosure, and adequate interventions to protect older persons from living in undignified conditions.

Strengthen Families and Their Preferred Sources of Support

As the most common first responders to dementia, it is critical to understand the needs of the individual within a context of how he/she is connected to their family network. While this is not universal for all South Africans, it highlights the need to deconstruct biomedical approaches that simply define person-centred care in isolation, when families often have complex hierarchies and customs that directly inform health decision-making and therefore the health outcomes of older people in need of care. For the majority of South Africans, person-centred approaches to biomedical treatment and care can be strengthened when including families in these discussions. Traditional healing has mastered these approaches, where families prefer their family-centred strategies to approach health needs within the family network. In this context, responding to a sick family member is therefore often a collective response, not an individual one. For these reasons, spiritual leaders (including religious and traditional leaders) are often the first port of call that provide families with spiritual and social 'first aid' when someone is ill. Traditional healers are therefore an untapped resource for providing information and support for dementia-related issues. Sharing knowledge between biomedical and spiritual/social resources provides a unique opportunity for South Africa to strengthen families and their preferred sources of support to respond in a coordinated way to combat stigma and provide the needed support for people with dementia and their families. This is especially true when considering family needs for accessible, cultural-friendly long-term care and support provisions.

Bridging Traditional and Biomedical Approaches

Historically, biomedical approaches and traditional healing have been polarised where traditional African medicine is often stigmatised as irrational and ungrounded in science (Sobiecki, 2014). Cultural prejudices and professional arrogance on both sides have created barriers to understanding the needs of families in South Africa and continue to fragment supportive and therapeutic responses to older persons and their families in need of guidance and care. Not discounting the history of harmful medicines and practices on both sides, it is important that health staff and traditional healers understand the full patient history, treatments received, and how these interact to affect the person with dementia. Concealing therapies out of fear or shame can have disastrous effects on the older person's health outcomes and underscores the need to bridge traditional and biomedical approaches if South Africa is going to strengthen its response to dementia in culturally acceptable ways. However, the challenge remains in bringing these worlds together to work towards common goals that include early detection, referral, and management of dementia to ensure quality of life and ageing with dignity. Genuine partnerships between biomedicine and traditional medicine are needed where knowledge exchange is bi-directional and finding common ground in identifying best practices to support families. While WHO has supported the use of scientifically proven traditional medicines for decades (Amazigo et al., 2010), it is important to note that not all differences between traditional healing and biomedicine can be reconciled as the former includes beliefs based on mysticism, superstition, deity, and supernatural abilities (i.e. witchcraft) (Sifuna, 2022). Common ground can, however, be found in the use of herbs and botanical remedies that have been used over the ages, for example, plants that have now gained scientific support for managing memory loss and debilitative mental disorders (Stafford et al., 2008), epilepsy (Marchetti et al., 2011), and anti-depressant like effects (Bonokwane et al., 2022). Ultimately, in the case of dementia, in an absence of a cure, the focus should be on preparing families for the prognosis of the condition and how best to prepare for the future.

Conclusion

Care pathways for dementia should ideally include culturally acceptable sources of support, where referrals to the biomedical and traditional routes are transparent and collaborative in providing holistic care for people with dementia and their families. These existing social and spiritual networks can be activated to help fill the gaps in existing dementia care and support provisions, through information sharing and awareness raising around issues of dementia in South Africa.

Trained traditional healers, together with trained general practitioners and primary healthcare staff (i.e. nurses, community health workers and allied health professionals), are largely under-used resources in South Africa for the identification, referral, and management of dementia. Capacity constraints within the healthcare setting need attention, especially considering that health systems often focus responses on safety through providing physical care at the expense of dignity in care (e.g. sitting down and spending time with the individual or the family) (Houghton et al., 2016; Jones et al., 2006). The role of traditional and indigenous belief systems in early identification, referral, and support also needs attention. Education on dementia should embrace broader understandings of illness and acknowledge the importance of spirituality in cultures to activate locally acceptable sources of support as potential allies in combatting the stigmatisation of dementia within communities. Decisions about the care and support for a family member with dementia largely rest within the family. Roles of providing care and support are often patriarchal and gendered, with women often necessitated to give up their participation in economic activities to provide full-time care to a family member with progressing care needs (Lloyd-Sherlock, 2019). When families are unsupported and caring for someone with dementia in isolation, risk of abuse is a reality often concealed or unreported. Care pathways for older persons should therefore be clear and unambiguous and provide access to all relevant sectors that include (and are not limited to) healthcare, social development, long-term care, civil society, as well as policing and the judicial system—that work harmoniously to respond to health and protection needs of older persons and prevent risk of abuse or secondary trauma.

For most South Africans, ageing is hard and an undignified experience when living in a context of poverty, inequality, and unemployment. Risk of abuse and exploitation creates unique vulnerabilities when older persons are targeted for their pensions and assets by strangers and family alike. Ageing in place with dignity cannot be achieved without addressing these social determinants of violence against older persons in South Africa and strengthening community-based responses for those who need healthcare, protection, and support. Families remain a critical support system to older persons and often are best placed to deliver this support. It is the absence of choice, training, and supplementary formal support that increase the likelihood of elder abuse. Ageing in place with dignity can only be achieved if the social structures older persons belong to (e.g. families and communities) are supported to facilitate positive health outcomes, safety, and improved quality of life for all South Africans.

References

Adewuya, A. O., & Oguntade, A. A. (2007). Doctors' attitude towards people with mental illness in Western Nigeria. *Social Psychiatry and Psychiatric Epidemiology, 42*(11), 931–936.

Ally, Y., & Laher, S. (2008). South African Muslim faith healers perceptions of mental illness: Understanding, aetiology and treatment. *Journal of Religion and Health, 47*(1), 45–56.

Alzheimer's Association. (2019). *Dementia: Symptoms, diagnosis, causes, treatments.* https://www.alz.org/alzheimers-dementia/what-is-dementia

Alzheimer's Disease International. (2024). *Importance of a timely diagnosis.* https://www.alzint.org/about/symptoms-of-dementia/importance-of-early-diagnosis/

Amazigo, U., Chatora, R., Diarra-, A. J., Lucile, N., Tigest, I., Matshidiso, K., Chris, M., Ngenda, M., Roungou, J.-B., Toure, B., Walker, O., Zielinski, C., Ajibola, S., Kouvividila, W., Mandzoungou, A., & Mavila, F. (2010). *The African health monitor.* World Health Organization, Regional Office for Africa.

Audet, C. M., Ngobeni, S., Graves, E., & Wagner, R. G. (2017). Mixed methods inquiry into traditional healer's treatment of mental, neurological and substance abuse disorders in rural South Africa. *PLoS One, 12*(2), 1–14.

Baharudin, A. D., Din, N. C., Subramaniam, P., & Razali, R. (2019). The associations between behavioral-psychological symptoms of dementia (BPSD) and coping strategy, burden of care and personality style among low-income caregivers of patients with dementia. *BMC Public Health, 19*(447), 1–12.

Benade, S. (2012). Support services for people suffering from dementia in the rural areas of Kwa-Zulu Natal, South Africa. *Dementia, 11*(2), 275–277.

Bonokwane, M. B., Lekhooa, M., Struwig, M., & Aremu, A. O. (2022). Antidepressant effects of South African plants: An appraisal of ethnobotanical surveys, Ethnopharmacological and phytochemical studies. *Frontiers in Pharmacology, 13*.

Campbell-Reay, A. M., & Browne, K. D. (2001). Risk factor characteristics in carers who physically abuse or neglect their dependants. *Aging & Mental Health, 5*(1), 56–62.

Cooper, C., Balamurali, T. B. S., & Livingston, G. (2007). A systematic review of the prevalence and covariates of anxiety in caregivers of people with dementia. *International Psychogeriatrics, 19*(2), 175–195.

De Jager, C., Msemburi, W., Pepper, K., & Combrinck, M. (2017). Dementia prevalence in a rural region of South Africa: A cross-sectional community study. *Journal of Alzheimer's Disease, 60*(3), 1087–1096.

Downes, C., Fealy, G., Phelan, A., Donnelly, N., & Lafferty, A. (2013). *Abuse of older people with dementia: A review*. National Centre for the Protection of Older People (NCPOP), University College Dublin.

Van Dyck, C. H., Swanson, C. J., Aisen, P., Bateman, R. J., Chen, C. C., Gee, M., Kanekiyo, M., Li, D., Reyderman, L., Cohen, S., & Froelich, L. (2023). Lecanemab in early Alzheimer's disease. *The New English Journal of Medicine, 388*(1), 9–21.

Farina, N., Jacobs, R., Turana, Y., Fitri, F. I., Schneider, M., Theresia, I., Docrat, S., Sani, T. P., Augustina, L., Albanese, E., Comas-Herrera, A., Du Toit, P., Ferri, C. P., Govia, I., Ibnidris, A., Knapp, M., & Banerjee, S. (2023). Comprehensive measurement of the prevalence of dementia in low- and middle-income countries: STRiDE methodology and its application in Indonesia and South Africa. *British Journal of Psychology Open, 9*(4).

Goergen, T., & Beaulieu, M. (2013). Critical concepts in elder abuse research. *International Psychogeriatrics, 25*(8), 1217–1228.

Government Gazette. (2006). *Older persons act (no. 13 of 2006)*, Vol. 13. The Presidency.

Houghton, C., Murphy, K., Brooker, D., & Casey, D. (2016). Healthcare staffs' experiences and perceptions of caring for people with dementia in the acute setting: Qualitative evidence synthesis. *International Journal of Nursing Studies, 61*, 104–116.

Jackson, S. L. (2016). All elder abuse perpetrators are not alike. *International Journal of Offender Therapy and Comparative Criminology, 60*(3), 265–285.

Jacobs, R., Schneider, M., & Farina, N. (2022a). *Elder abuse in South Africa: Measurement, prevalence and risk*. University of Cape Town.

Jacobs, R., Schneider, M., Farina, N., du Toit, P., & Evans-Lacko, S. (2022b). Stigma and its implications for dementia in South Africa: A multi-stakeholder exploratory study. *Ageing & Society, 44*, 1–31.

Jones, J., Borbasi, S., Nankivell, A., & Lockwood, C. (2006). Dementia related aggression in the acute sector: Is a Code Black really the answer? *Contemporary Nurse: A Journal for the Australian Nursing Profession, 21*(1), 103–115.

Jordan, C. (2009). *Older person's programme: Concept paper*. Western Cape Department of Social Development.

Kalula, S. Z., & Petros, G. (2011). Responses to dementia in less developed countries with a focus on South Africa. *Global Aging, 7*(1), 31–40.

Khonje, V., Milligan, C., Yako, Y., Mabelane, M., Borochowitz, K. E., & De Jager, C. A. (2015). Knowledge, attitudes and beliefs about dementia in an urban Xhosa-speaking community in South Africa. *Advances in Alzheimer's Disease, 4*, 21–36.

Kotzé, C. (2018). Elder abuse-the current state of research in South Africa. *Frontiers in Public Health, 6*, 358.

Lloyd-Sherlock, P. (2019). Long-term care for older people in South Africa: The enduring legacies of apartheid and HIV/AIDS. *Journal of Social Policy, 48*(1), 147–167.

Mahlathi, P., & Dlamini, J. (2015). *Minimum data sets for human resources for health and surgical workforce in South Africa's health system: A rapid analysis of stock and migration*. African Institute for Health and Leadership Development.

Marchetti, C., Gavazzo, P., Stafford, G. I., & Van Staden, J. (2011). South African plants used in traditional medicine to treat epilepsy have an antagonistic effect on NMDA receptor currents. *Journal of Ethnopharmacology, 137*(1), 382–388.

Mkhonto, F., & Hanssen, I. (2018). When people with dementia are perceived as witches. Consequences for patients and nurse education in South Africa. *Journal of Clinical Nursing, 27*(1–2), e169–e176.

Momtaz, Y. A., Hamid, T. A., & Ibrahim, R. (2013). Theories and measures of elder abuse. *Psychogeriatrics, 13*, 182–188.

Moon, A., & Benton, D. (2000). Tolerance of elder abuse and attitudes toward third-party intervention among African American, Korean American, and White elderly. *Journal of Multicultural Social Work, 8*(3–4), 283–303.

Mushi, D., Rongai, A., Paddick, S. M., Dotchin, C., Mtuya, C., & Walker, R. (2014). Social representation and practices related to dementia in Hai District of Tanzania. *BMC Public Health, 14*(1).

Nichols, E., Steinmetz, J. D., Vollset, S. E., Fukutaki, K., Chalek, J., Abd-Allah, F., Abdoli, A., Abualhasan, A., Abu-Gharbieh, E., Akram, T. T., Al Hamad, H., Alahdab, F., Alanezi, F. M., Alipour, V., Almustanyir, S., Amu, H., Ansari, I., Arabloo, J., Ashraf, T., & Vos, T. (2022). Estimation of the global prevalence of dementia in 2019 and forecasted prevalence in 2050: An analysis for the Global Burden of Disease Study 2019. *The Lancet Public Health, 7*(2), e105–e125.

Ofori-Atta, A., Cooper, S., Akpalu, B., Osei, A., Doku, V., Lund, C., & Flisher, A. (2010). Common understandings of women's mental illness in Ghana: Results from a qualitative study. *International Review of Psychiatry, 22*(6), 589–598.

Peden, M., McGee, K., & Krug, E. (2002). *Injury: A leading cause of the global burden of disease, 2000*. World Health Organization.

Pengpid, S., Peltzer, K., & Ramlagan, S. (2021). Prevalence and correlates of hazardous, harmful or dependent alcohol use and drug use among persons 15 years and older in South Africa: Results of a national survey in 2017. *African Journal of Primary Health Care and Family Medicine, 13*(1), 1–8.

Pillemer, K., Burnes, D., Riffin, C., & Lachs, M. S. (2016). Elder abuse: Global situation, risk factors, and prevention. *Strategies, 56*, 194–205.

Prince, M., Bryce, R., Albanese, E., Wimo, A., Ribeiro, W., & Ferri, C. P. (2013). The global prevalence of dementia: A systematic review and meta analysis. *Alzheimers and Dementia, 9*(1), 63–75.

Prince, M., Wimo, A., Guerchet, M., Ali, G., Wu, Y., & Prina, M. (2015). *World Alzheimer report 2015: The global impact of dementia: An analysis of prevalence, incidence, cost and trends*. Alzheimer's Disease International.

Quinn, N., & Knifton, L. (2014). Beliefs, stigma and discrimination associated with mental health problems in Uganda: Implications for theory and practice. *International Journal of Social Psychiatry, 60*(6), 554–561.

Rawat, A. (2012). Gaps and shortages in South Africa's health workforce. *Africa Portal Backgrounder, 31*, 1–8.

South African Human Rights Commission (SAHRC). (2015). *Investigating hearing into systemic complaints relating to the treatment of older persons*. SAHRC.

South African Pagan Rights Alliance (SAPRA). (2014). *Witch-hunts in South Africa*. https://www.paganrightsalliance.org/remember-their-names

Sifuna, N. (2022). African traditional medicine: Its potential, limitations and challenges. *Journal of Healthcare, 5*(1), 141–150.

Sobiecki, J.-F. (2014). The intersection of culture and science in South African traditional medicine. *Indo-Pacific Journal of Phenomenology, 14*(1), 1–10.
South African Government. (2017). *Socio-economic impact assessment system (SEIAS): Final impact assessment (phase 2): White paper on National Health Insurance*. Department of Planning, Monitoring and Evaluation.
Spitte, S., Maier, A., & Kraus, E. (2019). Awareness challenges of mental health disorder and dementia facing stigmatisation and discrimination: A systematic literature review from Sub-Sahara Africa. *Journal of Global Health, 9*(2), 020419.
Stafford, G. I., Pedersen, M. E., Van Staden, J., & Jäger, A. K. (2008). Review on plants with CNS-effects used in traditional South African medicine against mental diseases. *Journal of Ethnopharmacology, 119*, 513–537.
Statistics South Africa. (2019). *General household survey 2018*. Statistics South Africa.
Statistics South Africa. (2021). *Statistical release: Mid-year population estimates 2021*. Statistics South Africa.
United Nations. (2015). *World population prospects: The 2015 revision*. United Nations.
World Health Organization (WHO). (2002). *Active ageing: A policy framework*. WHO.
World Health Organization (WHO). (2016). *Elder abuse: The health sector role in prevention and response*. WHO.
World Health Organization (WHO). (2017). *Abuse of older people on the rise—1 in 6 affected*. WHO.
World Health Organization (WHO). (2018). *Elder abuse: Key facts*. WHO.
World Health Organization (WHO). (2019). *Dementia: Key facts*. WHO.

9

Older People's Perceptions and Use of Technology

Pranitha Maharaj, Shanaaz Dunn, and Sachin Sewpersad

Abstract Advancements in technology have contributed towards an improved quality of life for older people; however, minimal evidence is documented in the African context. This chapter aims to address this gap by exploring the use of technology among older people in Durban, South Africa. This study draws on data collected from 60 participants aged 60 years and older. The interviews reveal that most older people have access to at least one technological device, but utilisation remains relatively low. Those who use technology do so for entertainment or to stay informed. Social media is an important means to stay connected to friends and family. The findings of this chapter have important

P. Maharaj (✉) • S. Sewpersad
School of Built Environment and Development Studies, University of KwaZulu-Natal, Durban, South Africa
e-mail: Maharajp7@ukzn.ac.za; SewpersadS@ukzn.ac.za

S. Dunn
Developmental, Capable and Ethical State, Human Sciences Research Council, Durban, South Africa
e-mail: SDunn@hsrc.ac.za

P. Maharaj (ed.), *Navigating Ageing in South Africa*, Sustainable Development Goals Series, https://doi.org/10.1007/978-981-97-9088-3_9

implications for the inclusion of older people in the use and development of technological advancement, which can improve the quality of life of a rapidly ageing population.

Keywords Older people • Ageing • Social media • Technology • South Africa

Introduction

Over the last several decades, the world's population has not only increased in size but has also become significantly older. By 2050, older people will constitute approximately 17% of the global population, leading to an increased dependency on those of working age to accommodate for the social expenditure and services that are required by them (United Nations, 2023). Older persons constitute a small portion of Africa's current total population; however, this is changing rapidly (Rademeyer & Maharaj, 2020). Estimates indicate that the size of sub-Saharan Africa's older population will overtake that of all other global regions within the twenty-first century. By 2050, Africa's older population is projected to increase to 235 million, or approximately 9.3% of the total population on the continent (He et al., 2020). South Africa has one of the largest shares of older people in the southern African region. Between 2002 and 2022, South Africa's older population grew from around 3.3 million to 5.7 million (9% of South Africa's total population) with a 69.7% increase in the population of older people in this period (Solanki et al., 2019). As of 2020, there were approximately 5.43 million people aged 60 and older in South Africa (Statistics South Africa, 2020).

Many African governments have not adequately addressed the difficulties that accompany the process of ageing (Maharaj, 2013). Sub-Saharan Africa remains one of the world's poorest regions with a relatively large younger population, where more focus is given to them in comparison to older people (Aboderin & Beard, 2015). The region has made sizable progress in trying to address older people's vulnerabilities and securing their basic rights. However, despite these advances, older people in the continent are continually marginalised against wider efforts to achieve socio-economic development in the region (Rademeyer & Maharaj, 2020). In addition to this, ageing populations experience specific challenges, especially in terms of care and the means to support older adult's ageing-in-place and living independently. This is especially pronounced in the developing world, where many countries are experiencing rapidly ageing populations without the necessary fiscal investment or infrastructure in social services and healthcare (Woolrych, 2016). Thus, the relationship between ageing and technology has become more prominent in both the research field and public sector, and experts in these sectors believe that the challenges associated with the demographic shift to ageing populations can be bypassed using technological equipment (Pelizäus-Hoffmeister, 2016).

Technology may help promote a more active and healthier lifestyle, enhance safety, prevent social isolation and maintain the support network of the individual. It may also increase efficiency and effectiveness of health resources and social services (Woolrych, 2016). Technological advancement offers several opportunities for older people, such as increasing their autonomy, self-confidence and mobility by allowing them to 'age-in-place' by supporting healthcare and functional capabilities (Woolrych, 2016). The use of technology has been effective in improving access to information and enhancing communication. Communication technologies such as cell phones play a significant role in the daily lives of older people, especially in growing and maintaining their own network of relationships, thereby satisfying their social needs (Pelizäus-Hoffmeister, 2016). In a rapidly transforming society, older people are expected to adapt to new technologies (Roupa et al., 2010). However, they face difficulty in adapting to new technologies because of their lack of experience or physical restrictions caused by their current health status (Roupa et al., 2010). Older people may also require extra support for the independent management of their health, especially due to age-related conditions and loneliness. However, this is challenging due to their specific requirements (Dhillon et al., 2011). Technology-based health interventions such as telephonic healthcare, also known as telehealth or telecare, provide a channel for healthcare providers to deliver remote care and nursing services to patients in their homes (Dhillon et al., 2011).

Knowledge capabilities, as well as access and capacity to engage new technologies, are vital for successful development (Das & Drine, 2020). However, Africa faces barriers to technological advancement due to lack of infrastructure and capacity (Das & Drine, 2020). Currently, technology and ageing are progressively becoming intertwined, both as a result of active innovation policies and as a consequence of daily living; therefore, it is imperative to improve the theoretical understanding of the relationship between ageing and technology (Peine & Neven, 2021). The advancement of technology has significantly influenced the improvement of the lives of older people in several ways (Nierling & Domínguez-Rué, 2016).

In South Africa, traditional household structures are changing. An increase in urbanisation and migration has meant that many younger people have moved in search of better prospects, leaving fewer people to take care of older people, especially in rural areas (Maharaj, 2013). However, technological advances have allowed greater interaction between families and friends. The use of social media platforms, such as Facebook and WhatsApp, has also allowed older people to stay connected with others. Thus, the experience of ageing and socialisation is also shaped by technology. The increase in the use of technologies such as mobile devices offers a variety of new channels for reaching and communicating with older persons, such as delivering health-related messages and providing security or environmental hazard alerts via messaging services (Rademeyer & Maharaj, 2020). In the future, there will be a greater demand for more effective information and communication tools that guarantee the continued wellbeing of older people (Maharaj, 2020), thus highlighting the need for more research to be conducted and explored.

Further to this, the world is currently emerging from the deadly COVID-19 pandemic, and social media and technology have been playing a significant role in overcoming isolation as well as ensuring that people remain informed about prevention and protection from the spread of the virus throughout the world (Sathish et al., 2020). New mobile technologies and applications have been developed to fight the COVID-19 pandemic. These include tracking apps and chatbots that helped to reduce the spread of the virus by providing information and creating awareness to limit the impact on people, society, and organisations (He et al., 2021). Although various information and communication technologies (ICTs) have been developed to overcome the challenges of the pandemic, there is still an urgent need to better understand the roles of these ICTs, information systems and technology because they play an important role in an increasingly virtual era. In South Africa, the lack of access to internet-enabled devices and digital literacy, both of which are associated with poverty, are among the main barriers to accessing ICT devices and accessing the web (Gillwald et al., 2018). The more remote rural areas of sub-Saharan Africa have several challenges in accessing the internet due to a lack of finances and resources as well as limited infrastructure and internet connectivity challenges (Molawa, 2009). There are also further constraints to internet access, such as the lack of electricity, poor literacy levels and language barriers.

There are particular challenges in addressing how to support a higher quality of life for older people whilst developing solutions to reduce the healthcare and social costs of caring for older people, especially due to the rapidity at which populations are getting older (Woolrych, 2016). Since the 2000s, ageing populations have become the focus of extensive scientific and political discussions, and there are now multidisciplinary scientific approaches on the issues that come with them (Koch, 2010). However, there is not much research on the relationship between ageing and use of technology (Hoffman, 2022). Their influence on each other is also minimally documented; thus, this requires more research and insights as technology plays an important role in the daily lives of older people (Peine & Neven, 2021). It has become a much more salient part of the everyday lives of most people especially in terms of communication and access to information, and older people are no exception to this (Peine & Neven, 2021). The use of technology among older persons in Africa is a poorly studied topic that deserves greater attention, especially in an era of rapid change and technological advancement. Therefore, this chapter attempts to address this gap by focusing on use of technology among older people in Durban, South Africa.

Qualitative In-Depth Interviews

The study was conducted with older people living in Durban, located in the province of KwaZulu-Natal in South Africa. Durban has a population of approximately 3.5 million (Statistics South Africa, 2012). The city was chosen as the study area due to the cultural and demographic diversity of potential participants. There is also a large share of older people who reside in the province, more than 940,000 (Statistics South Africa, 2023). The study adopted a qualitative approach using a sample of older people in Durban, South Africa. Qualitative research targets data that cannot be measured in quantity, such as underlying motives, decisions, and desires, and primarily utilises in-depth interviews to obtain research data (Kothari, 2004). It is suitable for constructing and growing theories that may be related to personal experiences, perceptions and opinions of the participants in the study (Sloan & Quan-Haase, 2017). For this reason, a qualitative approach was best suited for this study in order to obtain detailed perspectives from older people about their use and access to technology.

There is no universal definition of an older person. Several countries often demarcate a person as being older at age 65 and older; nonetheless, this may be challenged by an increase in life expectancy, quality of life, and varying levels of functionality or capability (Sabharwal et al., 2015). In South Africa, older persons refer to all persons aged 60 years and older (Statistics South Africa, 2017). For this study, any person aged 60 years and above, who resided in Durban were eligible for participation in the study. In total, 60 interviews were conducted with men and women aged 60 years and older from various locations in Durban. Most of the participants (40) were Africans whereas non-Africans, which were inclusive of White, Coloured and Indian, were the minority in the study sample (20 out of 60). Most (17) were married, and fewer were either widowed (16), single (14), or divorced (3). The marital status of several participants (10) was undisclosed. Most participants had at least a secondary level of education, with a few who had only a primary school education and tertiary level of education.

Data was primarily collected using semi-structured interviews. The interview guide was broad and covered a range of aspects such as demographic characteristics, perceptions and opinions of technological devices, access to and use of certain technological devices, and the impact on their lives. Trained, bi-lingual fieldwork staff collected data from the study participants. The language of preference by the majority of older people was isiZulu. Both purposive and snowball sampling strategies were used as the study focused solely on a specific age group. Potential participants were identified by their eligibility criteria and were approached and informed about the nature and intent of the study.

Participants were informed that their identities would remain anonymous. They were assured that their names were not going to be used in the dissemination, instead identifiers were assigned to each participant. Participant identifiers were created by randomly assigning a number to each participant. They were required to provide consent for their participation in the study and interviews to be audio-recorded, either verbally or by signing an informed consent form. First, they were informed of the purpose and nature of the study and notified that their participation was voluntary. Participants were also informed that they were able to withdraw from the study at any given time, with no repercussions. Once the eligible participants agreed to partake in the study, interviews were arranged and conducted at their homes. Interviews lasted approximately 45 minutes and were recorded and transcribed verbatim in English for analysis and dissemination. The transcripts were thereafter analysed thematically by grouping, coding and counting similar responses in the data. Thematic analysis allowed responses to be arranged according to trends or patterns and systematically identify, organise and group information into patterns or themes in the data (Braun & Clarke, 2017).

Older People Navigating the Use of Technology

Studies suggest that older people are open to the use of technology because it improves their daily living and allows them to stay connected to family and friends (Koch, 2010; Peine & Neven, 2021). All the participants reported having access to some form of technological device.

However, the most commonly used devices were cell phones, television and radio. These devices make it easy for older people to stay in touch with family and friends. Two South African studies on technology use among older people found that receiving calls was the easiest and most visible advantage of the mobile phone among older people, while other features such as text messaging were perceived to be difficult and less useful (Chipps & Jarvis, 2017; Erasmus et al., 2022).

Participants mainly used cell phones (mobile phones), televisions, radios, telephones, tablets and computers, and older people use these devices for an array of reasons. It is not uncommon for older people to receive mobile phones as gifts. Consistent with other studies, this study found that they have become an important and indispensable part of their daily lives (Peine & Neven, 2021). The most prominent reason was to maintain contact with family and friends; thus, it was seen as a necessity. One older person explained: "*The phone helps me to communicate with my family, extended family. So, without it they would not be able to contact me*". Cell phones enable social interaction; it has allowed older people to remain socially connected. One study found that older people and other marginalised groups of the population tend to have better access and acceptance of mobile technology compared with other technologies (Gerber et al., 2010). It is common for older people to use mobile technologies as a means to stay connected to family and friends or keep informed about current affairs (Biniok et al., 2016).

Cell phones were also used for medical emergencies or when older people required financial assistance, especially among those who lived away from their families. One participant mentioned that they used it when they were alone at night and if they heard any strange noises, they would rely on it to alert others in the community about any incidents. In South Africa, crime is rife and older people are often targeted especially because they are vulnerable. They fear becoming victims of crime, especially since they may be living alone (Kasiram & Holscher, 2015).

> "Having a phone is extremely useful. For example, when there is an emergency, I can use my cell phone to call for an ambulance. If I hear disturbing sounds outside at night, I would call my neighbour and warn them, also you can communicate with other family members and ask about life".

Besides a cell phone, the use of a television was popular among many of the older people in this study. One older person, age 61 years, relies on her television as *"watching TV is the best way for me to relax"*. Most older people watched television to stay informed about current affairs, as noted by one man: "*I only watch news on the television I do not like all these other programmes. At the moment I do not have a radio*". However, they also do so for entertainment and religious programming as they believed that it allowed them to connect with their religion. One older person noted: "*I mostly watch the news; sometimes I watch church sermons and gospel music*".

The radio, a device no longer commonly used by younger people because of other advancements in technology, was used by a number of the older people in this study. This was mainly for the purposes of listening to music for entertainment. Although the radio is not a common device in many homes, most older people had access to one because they believed that "*it keeps you updated with everything happening around you*". The radio was also another means to stay informed about current affairs that are ongoing in the country. One 69-year-old explained: *"Yes, I listen to the radio … especially the News because they keep us updated about things that happen in our country"*. Some reported using the radio for other reasons. One older person mentioned that the information, which was available on the radio, was informative and helpful in maintaining a balanced and healthy lifestyle and diet. They mentioned that they used the radio to gain information on how to eat and keep healthy. A 65-year-old noted: *"I like listening to uKhozi FM because they are very informative. For example, they have a program about how to eat healthy and keep healthy"*.

Others debated the advantages of the television versus the radio. Some preferred the television to the radio. They believed that watching television provides insight into events and allows you to watch events as they unfold. However, with the radio, there is a need to visualise the event. For this reason, there was a strong preference for television over the radio.

> "I like TV because, of its visual images unlike the radio where you have to visualise everything. For example, if there is an accident somewhere in KwaNdengezi, TV will show me the visual images and I get to see the actual accident, but the radio will only report and we do not see the accident".

However, not all older people were in favour of the use of technological devices. Some felt that even though access and use of these devices did make a difference in their lives, they did not agree with the content that was broadcast, especially on the television. They felt that some of the content was explicit and included images of a sexual nature and children are exposed to this. Additionally, one participant believes that alcohol is advertised in an appealing manner and due to this, many of the youth indulge in its use.

> "In as much as these devices have a made a difference in our lives, I do not support a lot of things that are showcased on our TVs … now everything is out there, our children are exposed to all of these things, alcohol is sold on our TVs. When you see an alcohol advert you would believe it is not a drug, they sell it well and make it as appealing as possible, especially to the youth. And this has bad effects on our children".

Access to Internet and Social Media

The ability to use technology varies by older people's physical capacity and needs (Gell et al., 2015). The older participants were also asked if they had access to social media platforms such as WhatsApp and Facebook. Among participants who did have access to the internet and social media, the internet was mainly used for accessing Google or searching for jobs for family members. One participant, aged 68 years, stated that she used the internet to help her son search for job opportunities and used WhatsApp for sending and receiving messages, advertisements and media files to and from friends.

> "Internet, on my phone, I do. Sometimes, when my son is looking for job adverts or something, WhatsApp, it helps me. Say I want to forward a message, a picture or a video to someone, or if I need any of these from someone. For example, they can send me adverts of available jobs for my son or anyone who might need it".

Some were reliant on Google for information or providing answers to questions they may have. One participant, aged 64 years, mentioned that she did not go a single day without using the popular internet browser.

> "Yes, I do have WhatsApp and Facebook; we communicate with others there that are doing the same work as I am, so it really helps. Yes, I do have [internet] access, I do not go a day without using google, it helps me when I am not clear with maybe some cases then it gives me clarity and I can do it on my own. I do not need help".

Even though some of the participants accessed the internet and social media platforms, the majority of older people were not able to do so. Only a few of the participants had access to the internet, which contrasts with a study in the United States by Gell et al. (2015) which found that 47% of their study sample had access to the internet. This may indicate a disparity between internet access and use between more developed and developing nations. Of those who did have access to the internet, the majority were able to use it themselves, while others required some help from family members. A few participants had access to the internet yet did not make use of it because they were unaware of how to use it. The participants did not express any desire to access or learn how to use these smartphone platforms. This may be worrisome as the internet has an impact and positive influence on health education as ICTs may increase use of health care services, improve service delivery and enable older people to improve the management of their personal wellbeing (WHO, 2011). Gell et al. (2015) found that lower use of the internet was associated with higher levels of morbidity and increasing age as older people have greater limitations in their physical capacity to use these technologies due to higher levels of disability, vision impairment, and memory limitations. This suggests that people may be less likely to make use of the internet as they age.

The reasons for this included medical conditions that prevented prolonged use of the mobile phone, negative beliefs or notions of addiction that surround social media, and the lack of knowledge about the internet and social media platforms. Some of the older people suggested that they suffer from arthritis and, as a result, they cannot use their smartphone for a prolonged period.

> "No, as I have said, I have arthritis, which means I cannot type on WhatsApp because I have arthritis. I cannot keep pressing the phone and playing with it, I only listen to the radio and dial when having incoming calls or when I call".

Others were not in favour of social media because they felt that it is time consuming. Faye et al. (2016) found that the excessive use of social media such as WhatsApp has negative consequences such as losing interest in the real world, loss of control, serious interference in everyday life and constant dependence on the application. This is interesting to note, as one participant stated that they did not use social media such as WhatsApp due to their perception and fear that the messenger makes one '*stupid*' and felt that it caused children to '*lose their minds*'.

Others stated that they did not access the internet because they were unaware of its purpose. They only ever heard people talk about the internet and did not know what it was, nor did they have access to or use social media such as WhatsApp. This participant did not express the desire to access or learn how to use smartphone platforms.

> "Internet no, I only hear people speaking about it, I do not even know what it is. I only have a phone. I just use it for calls. I do not even have things like WhatsApp because I do not know how to use them".

It is not always easy for older people to learn how to use new technology; therefore, many rely on assistance from others; often from their children or grandchildren. The majority of older people who did use the internet suggested that they did not need assistance accessing the internet, while others required assistance from family members. Some suggested that although they have access to the internet, they did not utilise it for any purpose.

Advantages and Disadvantages of Technology

'I Think Technology Is Good'

Technology can undoubtedly serve as a means to improve the lives of older people in several ways (Nierling & Domínguez-Rué, 2016). Most older people suggested that technology improved their lives or made it easier in some way. They observed that they preferred technological advancements as it made their lives easier. It has also reduced the time it takes to go and physically meet other people. They can communicate without having to travel. Some of them also suggested that they would like to learn more about technology.

> "I think technology is good, although it has taken me some time to learn about it. I could learn more, but I think I'm getting by with just what I know".
>
> "I am happy, things were hard before you could not just have a conversation with someone who is in Johannesburg while you are in Durban in one day. This technology made our life much easier".
>
> "It has indeed made my life easier in terms of communication, I do not have to spend time travelling to reach people. We can easily communicate via the phone".

'You Can Get Addicted to It'

Some of the older people felt that there were some disadvantages to the use of certain devices. They believed that one becomes reliant on such devices for information and entertainment, and they do not want to do anything else, and as a result, it becomes addictive. One woman noted: "*You can get addicted to it where you do not want to do anything else you just want to watch [television]*". Some reflected on their experiences, arguing that they suffered from health complications because they used certain devices too often. For example, one participant explained that it strained her eyes, and therefore, she suffered from vision difficulties, and occasionally, this led to the experience of headaches. She explained: "*Well, the eyesight is not as good as before, you can strain the eye, and sometimes I get a headache*". Other participants stated that sometimes the broadcast content, such as that in soap opera television shows, is not appropriate for younger viewers. One woman gave her opinion, stating "*What I do not like about watching TV is sometimes the things they show in soap operas are unpleasant or not suitable to children*".

Other participants suggested that technology did not make a difference to their lives, while a few suggested that it made life more difficult. Only a few of participants stated that they preferred the era before the development of modern technological devices due to the complications associated with prolonged use.

> "Technology is a fantastic thing in this modern era, but I do not think that it is the greatest thing depending on the kind of control you have on technology … kids are going on to the cell phone and Googling things about sex and inappropriate things and inappropriate behaviour without even the parents monitoring them".

Although many older people had access to some technological devices, there are other devices which may be needed to improve their lives. Most participants suggested that they did not require any technological device to make their lives easier. One participant stated that they could not keep demanding assistance from their children to use the devices. Others also felt that it was difficult for them to learn how to use newer devices and that it would be a tedious process for them.

> "You see, we are old, we cannot keep asking things from the children. It is tiring, and I would not even know how to use these things".
>
> "No, I am old now. Technology is for you kids, the new generation".

Older people may often have difficulties in learning how to use new technologies due to lower cognitive ability or lack of skills at older ages (Roos & van Greunen, 2022; Roupa et al., 2010; Wu et al., 2019). Moreover, in cases where older people would like to learn, they may often have no means to do so as their children or grandchildren may be impatient in assisting them (Roos et al., 2022).

Those who did not have the commonly mentioned devices wished to possess them as a means to make their lives easier. Some of these devices included a cell phone to communicate with family, a geyser to ensure access to hot water and a tumble dryer to help with the laundry. One participant stated that even though they had a washing machine, a tumble dryer would be a great addition to their daily lives. Another participant stated that he would like to "*a home telephone*" as he believed "*that they do not use as much airtime as the cellphone*". For him, the call rates for landline phones are much cheaper than when using a cell phone.

Use of Technology in the Future

Living longer has become a possibility due to the increase in life expectancy over the last 150 years (Nierling & Domínguez-Rué, 2016). Recently, expectations of being independent and actively ageing at home have been used to describe and characterise healthy and successful ageing in Western societies (Mort et al., 2013). The interviews suggest that many older people use some form of technological device daily. However, the most used devices were cell phones, televisions and radios. These devices make it easy for older people to stay in touch with daily events. Older people used devices for various purposes. The television was mainly used for entertainment, to stay informed of current affairs and informative programming. Landline telephones and cell phones were mainly used for communication. Radios were mainly used for spiritual guidance and entertainment.

The study found that most older people did not have access to the internet or social media applications such as WhatsApp. In addition, some participants demonstrated a reluctance to learn more about social media or the internet for future use as they felt that they lacked the skill to use them. The fact that very few older people have access to or make use of these outlets is worrisome, as they are the most vulnerable to morbidity and mortality. The internet also provides regular updates on current developments, which may directly influence their lives.

> "No, I do not like things like WhatsApp because it is a new thing, and it only came now when I am old. My mind is not even that active so I cannot start now learning how it works and all that. With my little knowledge it is very hard to use all these things".

Some older people argued that technology made life more difficult. Research has suggested that older people may refuse to use any device if it is too complicated (Fernández-Ardèvol, 2016). It was also discovered that many of the older people observed that technology did not have any impact on their lives, while some wanted to learn more about using technology. Most older people saw technological devices as positively impacting their lives, and some felt that much has changed due to the improvements in technology. They agreed that "*things have changed for the better*". The participants further explain that some technologies, such as cell phones, make it much easier and more efficient to communicate than in the past which relied less on technological forms of communication, such as use of postal letters, which would take much longer to reach their destination.

> "We cannot go back to the past now, a lot has changed and going back there, to all the suffering, would not be good. Now you can even do everything sitting at home through these phones unlike our days when we wrote letters. You see if I were to choose between writing a letter, email, fax or call; I would just choose calling because it is way faster. Now imagine if I had to send a letter, how long it will take to go where I wanted it to go".

In the future, older people are projected to be more receptive and responsive to technology (Koch, 2010). Better knowledge of technology use among older people may help direct interventions that aim to improve the health and quality of life of ageing populations (Gell et al., 2015). Advancement in ICTs through the internet and mobile phones are renowned for their possible high impact on health education and health monitoring (WHO, 2011). It is therefore critical to invest in developing the skills of older people in using technology. This is especially in situations where older people show enthusiasm for learning how to use modern ICTs such as the internet and social media.

According to the International Telecommunication Union (ITU, 2021), it is imperative that now more than ever, older persons must be able to effectively use digital technologies. This is not only for their own health and welfare but also to communicate with family, keep abreast with the latest information and advice, and to help bypass feelings of isolation. Digital skills are very important; however, gaining them is more challenging for older people. The COVID-19 pandemic has highlighted the salience of having the essential digital skillsets to navigate a more virtual era and have access online (ITU, 2021). The 2030 Sustainable Development Agenda highlights 'leave no one behind' as one of its main goals, which seeks to promote the social, economic, and political growth and inclusion of all members of society, irrespective of their demographic background, including age (United Nations, 2016). An ageing population provides noteworthy opportunities for sustainable development and is related to the active participation and contribution of older persons in the economy, labour market and society (Dugarova, 2017). It is important to prepare for the economic and social transformations associated with ageing and old age in order to progress towards the implementation of the Sustainable Development Goals. This is imperative to ensure that the older population lead independent, healthy and productive lives, while empowering them to make their own decisions and choices in all aspects of their lives (Dugarova, 2017).

Conclusion

The study found that many older people have access to some form of technological device, mainly televisions, cell phones and radios. However, the use of technology remains low among older people. The findings of this study have important implications for ageing policies as technologies are prominently and continuously being advanced to solve the challenges presented by an ageing society. Society must prepare for changes associated with ageing in order to safeguard progression towards the implementation of the Sustainable Development Goals. To ensure that 'no one is left behind', all members of society must be included in broader efforts in the world's progression and transformation towards a more technological and digital age.

The scarcity of studies on ageing and technology in South Africa prompts the need for more research as the country's ageing population continues to grow. A larger, nationally representative survey can be administered to older people to gain key insights that are needed to enhance and promote the use of technology for improved quality of life. It is recommended that more in-depth research into accessibility, use, and functionality of technological innovations as a feasible intervention to assist with the problems of ageing is needed. Research on this will benefit the formulation, revision and implementation of existing policies and initiatives that surround ageing and technology. ICT support for older people can bring about a considerable number of benefits, such as assisting with factors such as patient diagnoses, treatment and health education. Service providers of telecare technology have been given positive feedback on its use for patient management, reporting improved relationships with and the monitoring of patients, and the potential for saving costs (Woolrych, 2016).

References

Aboderin, I. A., & Beard, J. R. (2015). Older people's health in sub-Saharan Africa. *The Lancet, 385*(9968), 9–11.

Biniok, P., Menke, I., & Selke, S. (2016). Social inclusion of elderly people in rural areas by social and technological mechanisms. In E. Domínguez-Rué & L. Nierling (Eds.), *Ageing and technology: Perspectives from the social sciences.* Transcript Verlag.

Braun, V., & Clarke, V. (2017). Thematic analysis. *The Journal of Positive Psychology, 12*(3), 297–298.

Chipps, J., & Jarvis, M. A. (2017). Technology-assisted communication in older persons in a residential care facility in South Africa. *Information Development, 33*(4), 393–405.

Das, G. G., & Drine, I. (2020). Distance from the technology frontier: How could Africa catch-up via socio-institutional factors and human capital? *Technological Forecasting and Social Change, 150,* 1–16.

Dhillon, J. S., Ramos, C., Wünsche, B. C., & Lutteroth, C. (2011). Designing a web-based telehealth system for elderly people: An interview study in New Zealand. In *24th international symposium on Computer-Based Medical Systems (CBMS)*. Piscataway.

Dugarova, E. (2017). *Ageing, older persons and the 2030 agenda for sustainable development*. United Nations Development Programme.

Erasmus, M., Bothma, E., & Roos, V. (2022). Developing a questionnaire to investigate older individuals' cell phone use and age-inclusive implementation through technology. In V. Roos & J. Hoffman (Eds.), *Age-inclusive ICT innovation for service delivery in South Africa: A developing country perspective*. Springer.

Faye, A. D., Gawande, S., Tadke, R., Kirpekar, V. C., & Bhave, S. H. (2016). WhatsApp addiction and borderline personality disorder: A new therapeutic challenge. *Indian Journal of Psychiatry, 58*(2), 235–237.

Fernández-Ardèvol, M. (2016). An exploration of mobile telephony non-use among older people. In E. Domínguez-Rué & L. Nierling (Eds.), *Ageing and technology: Perspectives from the social sciences*. Transcript Verlag.

Gell, N. M., Rosenberg, D. E., Demiris, G., LaCroix, A. Z., & Patel, K. V. (2015). Patterns of technology use among older adults with and without disabilities. *The Gerontologist, 55*(3), 412–421.

Gerber, T., Olazabal, V., Brown, K., & Pablos-Mendez, A. (2010). An agenda for action on global e-health. *Health Affairs, 29*, 233–236.

Gillwald, A., Mothobi, O., & Rademan, B. (2018). *The state of ICT in South Africa*. Research ICT Africa.

He, W., Aboderin, I., & Adjaye-Gbewonyo, D. (2020). *Africa aging: 2020*. United States Government Printing Office.

He, W., Zhang, Z. J., & Li, W. (2021). Information technology solutions, challenges, and suggestions for tackling the COVID-19 pandemic. *International Journal of Information Management, 57*, 102287.

Hoffman, J. (2022). 'Leapfrog technology': Locating older (South) Africans at the ICT interface. In V. Roos & J. Hoffman (Eds.), *Age-inclusive ICT innovation for service delivery in South Africa: A developing country perspective*. Springer.

International Telecommunication Union (ITU). (2021). *Technology and older persons: Ageing in the digital era*. International Telecommunication Union.

Kasiram, M., & Holscher, D. (2015). Understanding the challenges and opportunities encountered by the elderly in urban KwaZulu-Natal, South Africa. *South African Family Practice, 57*(6), 381–386.

Koch, S. (2010). Healthy ageing supported by technology–a cross-disciplinary research challenge. *Informatics for Health and Social Care, 35*(3–4), 81–91.
Kothari, C. R. (2004). *Research methodology: Methods and techniques*. New Age International.
Maharaj, P. (2013). Introduction. In P. Maharaj (Ed.), *Aging and health in Africa*. Springer.
Maharaj, P. (2020). Introduction. In P. Maharaj (Ed.), *Health and Care in old age in Africa*. Routledge.
Molawa, S. (2009). The "first" and "third world" in Africa: Knowledge access, challenges and current technological innovations in Africa. *First International Conference on African Digital Libraries and Archives (ICADLA-1).*
Mort, M., Roberts, C., & Callén, B. (2013). Ageing with telecare: Care or coercion in austerity? *Sociology of Health & Illness, 35*(6), 799–812.
Nierling, L., & Domínguez-Rué, E. (2016). All that glitters is not silver—Technologies for the Elderly in context. Introduction. In E. Domínguez-Rué & L. Nierling (Eds.), *Ageing and technology: Perspectives from the social sciences*. Transcript Verlag.
Peine, A., & Neven, L. (2021). The co-constitution of ageing and technology–a model and agenda. *Ageing & Society, 41*(12), 2845–2866.
Pelizäus-Hoffmeister, H. (2016). Motives of the elderly for the use of technology in their daily lives. In E. Domínguez-Rué & L. Nierling (Eds.), *Ageing and technology: Perspectives from the social sciences*. Transcript Verlag.
Rademeyer, S., & Maharaj, P. (2020). Patterns and trends. In P. Maharaj (Ed.), *Health and care in old age in Africa*. Routledge.
Roos, V., & van Greunen, D. (2022). Yabelana: Designing and introducing an age-inclusive and context-specific information and communication ecosystem. In V. Roos & J. Hoffman (Eds.), *Age-inclusive ICT innovation for service delivery in South Africa: A developing country perspective*. Springer.
Roos, V., Hoffman, J., & Oduaran, C. (2022). Intergenerational experiences around older persons' cell phone use in formal public domains. In V. Roos, J. Hoffman, V. Roos, & J. Hoffman (Eds.), *Age-inclusive ICT innovation for service delivery in South Africa: A developing country perspective*. Springer.
Roupa, Z., Nikas, M., Gerasimou, E., Zafeiri, V., Giasyrani, L., Kazitori, E., & Sotiropoulou, P. (2010). The use of technology by the elderly. *Health Science Journal, 4*(2), 118–126.
Sabharwal, S., Wilson, H., Reilly, P., & Gupte, C. M. (2015). Heterogeneity of the definition of elderly age in current orthopaedic research. *Springerplus, 17*(4), 516.

Sathish, R., Manikandan, R., Priscila, S. S., Sara, B. V., & Mahaveerakannan, R. (2020). A report on the impact of information technology and social media on Covid–19. In *Proceeding of the third International Conference on Intelligent Sustainable Systems (ICISS)*. Institute of Electrical and Electronics Engineers.

Sloan, L., & Quan-Haase, A. (Eds.). (2017). *The SAGE handbook of social media research methods*. Sage.

Solanki, G., Kelly, G., Cornell, J., Daviaud, E., & Geffen, L. (2019). Population ageing in South Africa: Trends, impact, and challenges for the health sector. In *South African health review 2019*. Health Systems Trust.

Statistics South Africa. (2012). *Census 2011 Municipal report—KwaZulu-Natal*. Statistics South Africa.

Statistics South Africa. (2017). *Mid-year population estimates 2017*. Statistics South Africa.

Statistics South Africa. (2020). *Mid-year population estimates 2020*. Statistics South Africa.

Statistics South Africa. (2023). *The social profile of older persons, 2017–2021*. Statistics South Africa.

United Nations. (2016). *Leaving no one behind: The imperative of inclusive development. Report on the world social situation 2016 executive summary*. United Nations.

United Nations. (2023). *World social report 2023: Leaving no one behind in an ageing world*. United Nations.

Woolrych, R. (2016). Ageing and technology: Creating environments to support an ageing society. *Geron, 15*(2), 66–70.

World Health Organization. (2011). *mHealth: New horizons for health through mobile technologies*. World Health Organization.

Wu, Y. H., Lewis, M., & Rigaud, A. S. (2019). Cognitive function and digital device use in older adults attending a memory clinic. *Gerontology and Geriatric Medicine, 5*, 1–7.

10

Navigating Transnational Identity: The Experience of Older Migrants

Sunday Israel Oyebamiji and Pranitha Maharaj

Abstract The chapter explores the social, economic and cultural challenges older migrants face in South Africa and their strategies for navigating these difficulties. It highlights the concept of transnationalism as central to understanding the identity of older migrants, with many maintaining strong connections to their home countries and influencing their social networks and economic strategies. These are examined by employing qualitative analysis combined with a comprehensive literature review. The interviews reveal that older migrants often experience significant barriers, including social isolation and cultural adaptation challenges. Despite these hurdles, they play a crucial role in bridging cultural gaps within their families and communities, acting as cultural mediators facilitating the transmission of heritage and values across generations. The chapter concludes by recognising and supporting the transnational

S. I. Oyebamiji (✉) • P. Maharaj
School of Built Environment and Development Studies,
University of KwaZulu-Natal, Durban, South Africa
e-mail: Oyebamijis@ukzn.ac.za; Maharajp7@ukzn.ac.za

P. Maharaj (ed.), *Navigating Ageing in South Africa*, Sustainable Development Goals Series, https://doi.org/10.1007/978-981-97-9088-3_10

identity of older migrants; South Africa can foster a more inclusive and diverse society that values the contributions of all its members.

Keywords Older migrants • Ageing • Culture • Adaptation • Transnationalism

Introduction

The global population is rapidly ageing, with significant implications for societies worldwide. As life expectancy increases and birth rates decline, the proportion of older adults is growing, reshaping demographics and challenging existing social structures (United Nations, 2019). The number of people aged 60 and over is expected to double by 2050, reaching nearly 2.1 billion globally (WHO, 2015). This demographic shift presents both opportunities and challenges, particularly concerning the well-being and social inclusion of older individuals.

Within the context of global migration, older people constitute a distinct yet often overlooked demographic group. While much attention is paid to younger migrants and their integration into new societies, the experiences of older migrants have been largely neglected. Older migrants face unique challenges related to ageing, mobility, and adaptation to new environments, which intersect with the complexities of transnational identity formation.

Alam (2023:34) defines transnational identity as a term that "generally applies to people who have cross-cultural living experiences between their home country and host countries". The concept is, therefore, relevant to this study because the work is about the cross-cultural experiences of older migrants in South Africa. Understanding this dynamic and identity among older migrants is essential for fostering social cohesion, promoting healthy ageing, and developing inclusive policies and services catering to their needs. By exploring the experiences of older migrants in South Africa, this chapter seeks to contribute to a deeper understanding of the transnational identity of older migrants, with a focus on their lived experiences.

At the intersection of population ageing and migration lie the experiences of older migrants, a population with unique needs and challenges. Older migrants comprise individuals who have relocated from their countries of origin to settle in new destinations, often in pursuit of economic opportunities, family reunifications, or asylum from conflict or persecution (Phillimore & Goodson, 2017). While migration offers the promise of new beginnings and opportunities, older migrants face distinct obstacles related to age, cultural adaptation and social integration (Phillimore & Goodson, 2017). Moreover, the process of ageing itself introduces additional complexities, including changes in health status, social networks and economic resources (WHO, 2022). Consequently, older migrants navigate a complex interplay of factors that shape their ageing experience in diverse cultural and social contexts, warranting specific attention in both ageing and migration studies.

The need for effective management of migration is attracting more attention and taking a new dimension globally; this is largely because no country has been able to isolate itself from the global migration trend, not even a country like South Africa, where many locals have openly demonstrated their resentment towards international migrants. It is also partly due to the existence of empirically established historical evidence that migration has been part and parcel of human culture since time immemorial (Oyebamiji, 2021). Therefore, the need for effective management and a new focus on policy formulation also requires new approaches. In this context, the chapter explores the experiences of migrants aged 60 years and older who have spent a good number of years, ranging from 10 to 20 years or more, in the host country.

In recent years, there has been increasing recognition of the significance of older migrants in the broader migration discourse. The ageing of populations in many developed countries has led to a growing demand for skilled labour and caregivers, prompting the inclusion of older individuals in migration patterns (Warnes et al., 2016). Older migrants, though often overlooked in migration studies, constitute a significant and unique subgroup with distinct motivations, challenges and contributions to the societies they settled in.

Amidst this new trend, South Africa has also emerged as an attractive destination for international migrants on the African continent (Crush

& Ramachandran, 2018; Oyebamiji, 2023). The country's rich cultural heritage, economic opportunities, and historical transformation from apartheid to democracy have drawn individuals seeking better prospects and improved livelihoods (Murray, 2019; Oyebamiji, 2023). Additionally, South Africa's geographical location and economic ties with neighbouring countries have positioned it as a regional hub, attracting migrants from diverse backgrounds (Crush et al., 2017).

Despite the growing presence of older migrants in South Africa, limited research has focused specifically on their experiences and challenges. Understanding the motivations behind their migration decisions, the ways in which they negotiate their cultural identities, the obstacles they encounter in accessing essential services, and the intergenerational dynamics that shape their lives within South African communities would be an asset in addressing their unique needs and in making them an instrument of social cohesion.

The chapter aims to fill this gap in the literature by exploring the experience of older migrants in South Africa amidst the dynamics of socio-cultural changes and their impact on transnational life. This is analysed with particular emphasis on the challenges they encounter and the nature of their responses. By focusing on the complexities and nuances faced by older migrants, this study shed insights into migration, ageing and transnationalism. Migrants face barriers in different ways. By virtue of their experience, older migrants are in a position to learn from such barriers, partly by examining the social context and taking a practical look at historical trends (United Nations, 2019).

Literature Review

Literature on international migration and ageing has seen substantial growth in recent years as researchers and policymakers recognise the significance of older migrants in shaping societies worldwide. The motivations behind international migration among older individuals are multifaceted and differ from those of younger migrants.

A review of the literature suggests that there are many reasons for migration. Economic factors, including the search for employment opportunities and better living standards, have been found to be less prominent among older migrants (Bollini & Siem, 2015). Instead, family reunification, especially in cases where adult children or relatives have settled in the destination country, emerges as a key motivation (Lynnebakke & Aasland, 2022). This familial dimension of migration decisions among older individuals plays a significant role in shaping their experiences in the host country.

Transnational ties play a crucial role in shaping the experiences of older migrants. Levitt and Jaworsky (2007) emphasise that older migrants often maintain strong connections with their countries of origin, engaging in transnational practices such as remittances, communication with family members, and participation in cultural and religious activities. These transnational ties contribute to the preservation of their cultural identities in the host country (Alarcón & Hinojosa, 2017). The negotiation between the maintenance of cultural traditions from their home country and adaptation to the new cultural context in South Africa becomes a defining aspect of older migrants' experiences.

Older migrants face unique challenges in South Africa in accessing essential services and support systems. Healthcare and well-being present significant obstacles, as older migrants may encounter language barriers, difficulties navigating the healthcare system and limited access to culturally appropriate healthcare services (Bollini & Siem, 2015). Employment opportunities are also often limited, particularly for older individuals with specific skill sets. Moreover, social support systems can be challenging to establish, especially for those with limited family networks in the host country (United Nations, 2019).

Despite these challenges, older migrants also bring valuable contributions to the host society. Their experiences and skills can be harnessed to address labour shortages and contribute to economic development (Warnes et al., 2016). Additionally, older migrants can enrich South African communities by sharing their diverse cultural backgrounds and fostering intercultural understanding (Crush et al., 2017).

The literature reveals the complexities of the experiences of older migrants in South Africa, highlighting their motivations, challenges and contributions in the context of international migration. The negotiation of transnational and cultural identities emerges as a central aspect of their experience. Policymakers and service providers need to consider the unique needs of older migrants to develop inclusive policies and support systems that foster their successful integration and well-being in South Africa.

Interviews with Older Migrants in South Africa

Migrants constitute a significant proportion of the global ageing population. Many moved from their home countries when they were much younger and now are ageing in their host countries. The chapter adopted a qualitative approach, allowing for an in-depth exploration of the experiences of older migrants in South Africa. Semi-structured interviews were utilised to collect data from a diverse group of older migrants representing a range of countries of origin and migration histories.

A qualitative methodology is well-suited to gain in-depth insights into the complexities and nuances of older migrants' lives, their motivations, challenges and contributions in the context of international migration (Denzin & Lincoln, 2018). By using qualitative methods, this study sought to capture the subjective experiences and perspectives of older migrants, allowing for a rich and contextual understanding of their lives in South Africa.

A purposive sampling strategy was used to select participants for this study. The sample consists of older migrants from diverse regions of the world, representing various countries of origin and migration histories. The inclusion of participants from varied backgrounds allowed for the exploration of the intersectionality of migration experiences and how cultural, social, and economic factors influence their lives in South Africa. In-depth interviews provide an opportunity to explore the personal narratives, motivations, and challenges faced by older migrants in a one-on-one setting.

Thematic analysis was employed to analyse the qualitative data gathered from interviews. This approach involves identifying patterns and themes within the data, allowing for the organisation and interpretation of the diverse experiences and perspectives of older migrants (Braun & Clarke, 2006). The analysis process involves iterative readings of the data, coding, and thematic categorisation to identify key findings and recurring patterns in the participants' narratives.

The Concept of Active Ageing

Active ageing is a multidimensional concept, primarily defined as "the process of optimising opportunities for health, participation, and security in order to enhance the quality of life as people age" (WHO, 2002). This concept is particularly pertinent when examining the experiences of older migrants in South Africa, a country marked by both its historical legacy of migration and its contemporary socio-economic challenges.

For older migrants, active ageing involves navigating a complex interplay of health, social participation and economic security. Health is a cornerstone of active ageing, yet older migrants often face significant barriers in accessing health care services. These barriers include language differences, lack of familiarity with the healthcare system, and, in some cases, xenophobia or discrimination from service providers (Moyo, 2018). This is what Pastor Moses from Nigeria meant by '*rejections*' and concluded that "*the reason for the rejection from the locals is ... that having come out of situations in Africa*", they "*now feel that you have come to take from them, which is not the case*". Older migrants from Africa are particularly fearful because they feel that they are blamed for the social ills that exist in the country. Consequently, their ability to maintain physical and mental health, a key aspect of active ageing, is compromised.

Participation, another critical component of active ageing, is influenced by social inclusion and community engagement. Older migrants in South Africa often experience social isolation due to cultural differences and separation from their extended families and home communities. However, those who manage to integrate into local communities or form networks with other migrants can find opportunities for meaningful participation. Such engagement can range from community volunteering to involvement in local religious or cultural organisations, which helps in maintaining their social and cognitive functions (Maharaj, 2013).

Economic security, the third pillar of active ageing, is particularly precarious for older migrants. Many migrants face challenges in securing stable employment due to their age, lack of formal education, or recognition of their qualifications. For this reason, Tamari, a woman from Zimbabwe, said, "*When it comes to the job, you know the job very well, but because you are not a South African, you are still discriminated against*". As a result, many migrants have to find employment outside of the formal sector. However, the informal nature of much of their employment means they lack access to pensions or social security benefits, heightening their financial vulnerability (Crush & Tawodzera, 2014). This economic insecurity directly affects their ability to live independently and maintain a satisfactory quality of life.

The socio-political environment in which they find themselves further complicates the active ageing process for older migrants. Policies and attitudes towards migrants can be restrictive and hostile, exacerbating their marginalisation and limiting their access to resources necessary for active ageing (Dodson, 2010). This is what one older woman, Tamari, meant in her assessment of the policy framework from the South African context, with particular emphasis on the permit, concluding that "*policymakers should see the impact of this [policy] on the people affected because this is causing problems for many Zimbabweans who are highly skilled who came through*" the Zimbabwean Exemptional Permit (ZEP). Similarly, in responding to this, a Ghanaian man said, "*When I came here, it was much easier for non-South Africans who acquired South African citizenship, but now there is a lot of politics, including xenophobia*". However, some initiatives exist to support older migrants, advocating for their rights and providing essential services which contribute positively to their ageing experience.

While the concept of active ageing provides a framework for enhancing the quality of life for older individuals, its application to older migrants in South Africa reveals significant challenges. Health disparities, social isolation, economic insecurity and systemic discrimination hinder their ability to age actively.

Place Identity, Place Dependence and Place Attachment

The intricacies surrounding the theories of place identity, place dependence and place attachment are key issues in psychology (Nisa et al., 2020), while the practical aspects of the concepts have engaged the attention of scholars and analysts in migration studies since the beginning of this century. This is because the concepts apply to humans as rational beings, and it is found that they constitute an essential ingredient in analysing and portraying the migration experience of individuals or groups in their host countries with particular emphasis on place and identity negotiation in the context of expected benefits from host and home countries and other places of interest to the migrant (Sieng & Szabo, 2023).

For older migrants, the issues of place identity, place dependence and place attachment constitute a major focus in the post-migration journey of life. This is because the reality of life becomes more glaring to the individual, and psychologically, there is the tendency to feel that the acquisition of material wealth alone may not provide true satisfaction and fulfilment. This is, in a way, reflected in the responses to the question, "*If you could go back to your home country, would you?*" The answers are in the affirmative, signifying the choice of their home countries for place identity, while South Africa satisfies the purpose of place dependence as they depend on the host country to build a career and earn a means of living. For the migrants, both host and home countries are important for this reason. This is why Sieng and Szabo (2023) posit that place identity and dependence are complementary in the life of older migrants since the identity affiliation to their country could not prevent them from embarking on migration to another country which possesses the enabling environment that they can depend upon to live a fulfilled life.

In South Africa, even though this set of migrants believe in return migration if they have the opportunity, they still believe strongly in the host country for place dependence and have enough reasons to continue living in the host country. However, one of the participants is reluctant to accept the offer of return migration even if there are positive developments that can make the home country serve the purpose of both place identity and place dependence. Thus, Adrienne from the United Kingdom said:

> Well, we love our life here and have been very happy. Still, with the current situation in the country and, particularly, the current situation, security is important to us. If crime increases, we might be tempted to go back to countries likely to favour us, but at the moment, we are not thinking about that. I think I settled in very quickly. As soon as I came from the UK, South Africa became my home. Having my family and grandchildren has made me happy. My family is here with me, and I think the older you are, the more you need family. Your children and grandchildren are there to support you. From my point of view, it is a great part of happiness that they are all here.

On the issue of place attachment, this study of older migrants in South Africa portrays some element of deviation in that we can only talk of partial place attachment from the responses and attitudes of the migrants. However, while this may be accommodated by a model of the place identity, dependence and attachment theory that tends to identify different degrees of attachment (Lynnebakke & Aasland, 2022), the issue of compulsory 'emotional bond' emphasised in traditional studies of the theme (e.g., Hidalgo & Hernandez, 2001; Lewicka, 2010), is not captured. Thus, the participants' responses contradict the theoretical conception of place attachment as the emotional intent and love that binds one to a particular community or environment.

In the aspect of place identity, most migrants pick their home country. Therefore, psychologically, South Africa only occupies the position of place dependence in their profile. All the migrants are attached to South Africa since this is where they have built their careers and earn a means of living. But this place attachment may be involuntary and, therefore, partial since all, with the exception of one, explained the barriers to migrants' visions and career development efforts arising from the hostile attitudes of many locals, including those who feel that migrants are obstacles to the creation of job opportunities in different ways as well as hindrances to the expansion of businesses in the informal economy. Thus, Moses, a man from Nigeria, said that "*this is why South Africans are hostile*". Along this line, Tamari, a woman from Zimbabwe, also noted that her staying in South Africa as a migrant made her realise that people are not as friendly as her country of origin. She had experienced discrimination because of her migration status and felt that it was unfair that opportunities arose because of social networks rather than expertise.

> When it comes to the job, you know the job very well, but because you are not a South African, you are still discriminated against and getting into other opportunities depends on who you know.

Oliver, a man from Zimbabwe, talks about his concerns about crime and xenophobia. In South Africa, there is the commonly held perception that migrants take jobs and women away from locals, and he was concerned about this worrying trend that is very widely supported.

> When you have lost a laptop before, for example, your laptop was stolen from the car's boot, those things worry me. Obviously, they talk about taking jobs and women. Those misconceptions must be dealt with. There have not been any studies that show that migrants are taking jobs from the locals.

What we refer to as 'involuntary and partial place attachment' in this study is better understood from the perspective of observation in psychology that place attachment may depend on the benefit derived by individuals from a community even when they have no emotional interest in the place (Inalhan et al., 2021). We can, therefore, talk of voluntary and impartial place attachment if the host country is able to create an environment that enables the immigrant to develop emotional love (i.e., place identity) in addition to serving the purpose of place dependence. However, from the responses, this is not easy to actualise in the South African context. Thus, Moses from Nigeria said:

> To be honest, my only problem is that they do not allow you to maximise your potential in the land. This is in the sense that once they see that you want to give your best, there is that kind of pressing you down. The case is different in Nigeria because they welcome foreigners and want to see what you can offer the land.

Similarly, Tamari from Zimbabwe said:

> Xenophobia makes me unhappy with South Africa. You can see that there are differences in treatment here. I am here because I have already brought up two boys here in South Africa, and those boys only know South Africa as home but they are told to go back to Zimbabwe.

Migrants only have a partial attachment to their home countries since the home country cannot meet all their life expectancies, including careers. Therefore, they are unable to play the total role of place dependence. However, this can be said to be voluntary because there is emotional interest or love behind it. This voluntary and emotional attachment is best reflected in the view of Oliver from Zimbabwe, who said, "*It has been good years*" in South Africa "*and very good hospitality, but home is home*". Similarly, Kofi from Ghana said, "*Nothing stops me from going back home; home is home*". However, it is not a complete attachment since the attachment is shared between the host (place of dependence) and the home country (place of identity).

However, in the South African context, the analysis is hardly complete without understanding the 'person', that is, individual emotional and psychological inclination in relation to the actualisation of life-long visions. This is followed by the 'process', which is the journey towards realising what WHO refers to as value life goals, and then the 'place', which refers to the community or environment the migrant derives inspiration from regarding identity and dependence.

The Person-Process-Place

The person-process-place (PPP) framework is commonly used in various fields such as organisational behaviour, psychology, urban planning and design thinking to understand the interplay between individuals, the processes they engage in, and the environments in which these interactions occur.

Scannell and Gifford (2014) and Inalhan et al. (2021) employed the concept of 'the person-process-place' (PPP) in the analysis of workplace attachment. These writers developed the model to explain the psychological and behavioural intricacies encountered when attachment has to do with the individual's assigned places of work. But at the transnational level, the PPP relationship also provides a platform for understanding certain trends and analysing some problems in migration. This is particularly helpful in exploring the experience of older migrants because, in a way, they are already made, and their migration life is already defined.

In the South African context, the migrant referred to as 'the person' in this model has a psychological and emotional experience derived from xenophobia and its attendant limitations or hazards. This is reflected in the viewpoints of the participants. All have one thing or the other to say about this. Thus, commenting on this, participant Tamari from Zimbabwe said:

> The biggest challenge is xenophobia! Nigerians can also testify to what I am saying. Because the locals are saying, Zimbabweans and Nigerians are taking their jobs. People think that migrants are coming to take their jobs.

For the older migrants in South Africa, what is referred to as 'the process' above embraces a host of issues in social life that are polarised by both local and external influences. In the host country, the process of getting there and sustaining the trend till old age involves managing different social contexts. Some of these are polarised with crisis, xenophobic violence and crimes. However, since the home country often serves as a place of identity for most migrants in a hostile host community, the home country's worldview, values and cultural milieu are among the factors at play when going through the process. At the same time, international agencies, for example, WHO, United Nations High Commission for Refugees (UNHCR), International Labour Organization (ILO), International Organization for Migration (IOM), and International Centre for Migration Policy Development (ICMPD) are setting standards that must be adhered to globally by all migrants, and these have far-reaching influence in defining the process. These are, therefore, essential issues to the older South African migrant even though he or she is retiring from active social life. In the host country, the process of getting there and sustaining themselves till old age involves managing different social contexts.

In most other parts of the world, the term 'place' is synonymous with the host country (Afshar et al., 2017; Sieng & Szabo, 2023). However, in the South African context, it is a complex issue, and it is reflected in the participants' responses. In this context, a place is not a single space for many migrants; sometimes, it could be two or even more. Thus, a participant from Kenya expresses himself directly when he talks of partial place dependence and why the original place identity in the home country provides the propelling inspiration and psychological vigour to endure hazards in the host country since there is still hope elsewhere, a place to be welcomed in case of return migration.

Responding to the question, "*How have you adapted to life in South Africa?*" Moses from Nigeria, said that "*it was pretty challenging to start with because the greatest shock*" is that when he was in Britain, he never experienced discrimination on account of his nationality. Thus, the concept of 'place' to older migrants in South Africa is instrumental to the analysis, having acquired experience gathered through a long history polarised by social crisis, in addition to rejections by locals. There are, therefore, a host of contradictions in trying to define what constitutes real place attachment as migrants. Unlike the young migrants, they refuse to be carried away by emotion, as the reality has been defined by a long history of events antithetical to the glamour visualised in the early years of arrival as a migrant.

Adaptation: Older Migrants and South African Lifestyle

The migration of older individuals to South Africa presents a fascinating dynamic between their established cultural identities and the new lifestyle they encounter. This integration process involves significant adaptation challenges influenced by various social, economic, and health factors. Understanding the experience of older migrants in South Africa requires a nuanced exploration of how they navigate these challenges and embrace their new environment. The process involves a host of issues, though the migrants believe in the actualisation of their expectations. For this reason, Mike from the United Kingdom feels it should be examined from both "*the positive and the negative aspect*" for objectivity and proper understanding of the entire scene.

One of the primary areas of adaptation involves the social integration of older migrants. Upon arrival, these individuals often face the daunting task of establishing new social networks. The loss of familiar social support systems from their countries of origin can lead to feelings of isolation and loneliness (Manzoni & Rolfe, 2019). Building new relationships in a different cultural context requires significant effort and time, often complicated by language barriers and diverging social norms. Moreover, participation in community activities can be hindered by age-related health issues, further impacting their ability to form meaningful connections.

Economic adaptation is a crucial aspect for older migrants in South Africa. Many older migrants face financial insecurity, as they might have limited access to pension schemes or social security benefits in their new country (Williams, 2018). The cost of living in South Africa, coupled with potential difficulties in securing employment due to age discrimination, can exacerbate economic challenges. Such discrimination is partly related to what Mike, from the United Kingdom, refers to as the "*misconception that migrants take South African jobs*" whereas "*migrants do the jobs that South Africans don't want or they don't have the skills to handle*". Consequently, some older migrants might become financially dependent on family members, adding another layer of complexity to their adaptation process.

Health and access to healthcare services are pivotal in the adaptation of older migrants. The South African healthcare system presents both opportunities and challenges for these individuals. On the aspect of opportunities and virtue of the system, Oliver, a Zimbabwean, explains some preferential benefits he enjoys in the health system, stating that "*my age has given me that opportunity*". This implies that older migrants receive due attention if the services are readily available. While there are state-funded health services available, the quality and accessibility of these services can vary significantly (Govender et al., 2020). Older migrants sometimes need to navigate a new healthcare system, which can be particularly challenging if they are unfamiliar with the language and procedures. This is more so as the stress associated with migration and adaptation can exacerbate pre-existing health conditions, making timely and effective healthcare even more critical.

Cultural adaptation plays a significant role in the lives of older migrants. South Africa's diverse cultural landscape offers a unique environment for migrants to explore and integrate new cultural practices. This has its own virtue that some older migrants have been able to utilise. Thus, a migrant research analyst from Ghana said, "*I have adapted quite well*". However, others identified a number of hurdles encountered during the process. Therefore, the process is not without its challenges. Adapting to new cultural norms while retaining their cultural identity can lead to a complex interplay of assimilation and preservation (Bhugra & Becker, 2005). A few older migrants, such as Moses from Nigeria and Tamari from Zimbabwe, find solace in cultural enclaves and religious norms through which they can connect with others from their home country, providing a sense of continuity and community.

The issue of lifestyle and adaptation is broad because it embraces both social conventions. At the same time, it varies from state to state and from region to region. Therefore, in South Africa, older migrants tend to approach the issue from a liberal perspective, especially as some components of lifestyle and adaptation depend on an area's climate and weather conditions. Adaptation is much easier if there are job opportunities available. Responding to this, Adrienne from the United Kingdom said: "*My career opportunity was good because I was a bit younger, and I had a wonderful job opportunity at a private school, so I stayed there for the rest of my teaching life. I will say that my age and career made me adapt well to life in South Africa*". Adaptation is influenced by the nature of social institutions as well as similarities in cultural practices. One participant from Ghana noted cultural similarities between his home country and the host country, arguing, "*they refer to bride price here as lobola; we pay it in Ghana too. It is just that it is not as expensive in Ghana as in South Africa*". There are also differences in cultural practices that have made adaptation more challenging. This is clear in the response of Oliver from Zimbabwe, who notes, "*our own culture is a little bit more conservative. In South Africa, their own is more liberal; children can sometimes do as they wish in the sense of control*".

Other respondents felt that there are a host of issues that influence adaptation. Mike from the United Kingdom notes that there are a number of factors that make South Africa a favourable destination for migrants. He explains, "*I think one of the reasons South Africa is desirable for people is the coastal sunshine, good lifestyle, and the low cost of living, which is very positive*". However, there are also numerous challenges facing the country which impact the situation of migrants, as he explains that "*the crime rate overseas is generally much lower. The other thing to bear in mind is the difference in unemployment rate, which we know is very high here*". Some migrants noted that adaptation is becoming increasingly more difficult as they are faced with increasing crime in the country. Reflecting on his journey, one participant from Ghana said: "*I will say I have adapted fairly well ... certain things shock me, though. Before 1994, it was not very bad. One thing I am still struggling with is the crime. Crime here is very bad; it is not as if there was no crime in West Africa, but there is more crime here in South Africa*". Another respondent has come to understand that adaptation may also involve a good level of tolerance. In the host country, migrants have to assimilate, and this requires leaving behind norms and traditions that they embraced in their home country, but now they have to adapt to the host country.

Adaptation is enhanced by healthy ageing, a component of active ageing. Therefore, the active ageing theory is used to explain the issue of adaptation from the perspective of older migrants. Understanding healthy ageing in relation to adaptation and within the context of the active ageing theory is significant as it has been observed that "many national strategic efforts have not focused on the health and well-being of older migrants, which is important to ensure that all people in the country maintain good health, improved quality of life, and independent living in old age, irrespective of their migrant status" (Zihindula et al., 2023). Besides, issues involving older migrants in the African context have been relatively sidelined in policy formulation and strategic planning in addition to the fact that this set of migrants is often vulnerable to poverty due to the absence of a well-structured social and public funding facility to control anticipated financial crisis among members of the group (Groth et al., 2019; Zihindula et al., 2023).

Overall, the adaptation of older migrants to the South African lifestyle is a multifaceted process influenced by social, economic, health and cultural factors. The successful integration of these individuals requires supportive policies and community initiatives that address their unique needs. By fostering an inclusive environment that values the contributions and experiences of older migrants, South Africa can enhance their quality of life and ensure their successful adaptation.

Conclusion

The experiences of older migrants in South Africa present a rich tapestry of challenges and opportunities that are deeply intertwined with their transnational lives. As they navigate their new environment, older migrants bring a wealth of cultural heritage and lived experiences that contribute to the multicultural fabric of South African society. Their journeys are shaped by various factors, including economic necessity, the pursuit of familial reunification, and the quest for safety from political or social unrest in their countries of origin. The study has demonstrated that an understanding of the perspectives and experiences of older migrants, including their response to new concepts in migration like place identity, place dependence and place attachment, is relevant to the creation of a new policy focus in migration to cope with the dynamics emanating from the rapidly changing socio-economic structures at both the global and national level.

Transnationalism is central to understanding the experiences of older migrants. Many maintain strong ties with their countries of origin, contributing to a dynamic interplay between their home and host countries. These transnational connections influence their identity, social networks and even economic strategies. For some, return migration becomes a viable option as they seek to reintegrate into their home countries after spending significant time in South Africa. However, this process comes with its own challenges, including readjustment to the home culture and reconnecting with family and friends. Future research could expand the scope to explore the experiences of specific subgroups of older migrants, such as refugees or those with distinct socio-economic backgrounds. Longitudinal studies may offer insights into the evolving nature of transnational identities and the long-term impact of policy interventions on older migrants' lives.

References

Afshar, P. F., Foroughan, M., Vedadhir, A., & Tabatabaei, M. G. (2017). The effects of place attachment on social well-being in older adults. *Educational Gerontology, 43*(1), 45–51.

Alam, F. (2023). *What is transnational identity?* Proceedings of the conference: Transnational crisis of people who go abroad. Transnational Press.

Alarcón, R. D., & Hinojosa, R. (2017). Transnational ageing and mental health: An overview. *The American Journal of Geriatric Psychiatry, 25*(9), 950–951.

Bhugra, D., & Becker, M. A. (2005). Migration, cultural bereavement and cultural identity. *World Psychiatry, 4*(1), 18–24.

Bollini, P., & Siem, H. (2015). No real progress towards equity: Health of migrants and ethnic minorities on the eve of the 21st century. *Social Science & Medicine, 41*(6), 819–828.

Braun, V., & Clarke, V. (2006). Using thematic analysis in psychology. *Qualitative Research in Psychology, 3*(2), 77–101.

Crush, J., & Ramachandran, S. (2018). Migration and South Africa's demographic dilemma. *Migration Policy Practice, 8*(4), 6–15.

Crush, J., & Tawodzera, G. (2014). Medical xenophobia and Zimbabwean migrant access to public health Services in South Africa. *Journal of Ethnic and Migration Studies, 40*(5), 655–670.

Crush, J., Tevera, D., & Chikanda, A. (2017). South-South migration and the labour market: The impact of the Lesotho–South Africa remittances corridor. *Urban Studies, 54*(4), 903–923.

Denzin, N. K., & Lincoln, Y. S. (2018). *The SAGE handbook of qualitative research* (5th ed.). Sage.

Dodson, B. (2010). Locating xenophobia: Debate, discourse, and everyday experience in Cape Town, South Africa. *Africa Today, 56*(3), 2–22.

Govender, V., Fried, J., Birch, S., Chimbindi, N., & Cleary, S. (2020). Disability Grant: A precarious lifeline for HIV/AIDS patients in South Africa. *BMC Health Services Research, 20*, 1–13.

Groth, H., May, J. F., & Turbat, V. (2019). Policies are needed to capture a demographic dividend in Sub-Saharan Africa. *Canadian Studies in Population, 46*(1), 61–72.
Hidalgo, M. C., & Hernandez, B. (2001). Place attachment: conceptual and empirical questions. *Journal of Environmental Psychology, 21*, 273–281.
Inalhan, G., Yang, E., & Weber, C. (2021). *Place attachment theory*. Routledge.
Levitt, P., & Jaworsky, N. B. (2007). Transnational migration studies: Past developments and future trends. *Annual Review of Sociology, 33*, 129–156.
Lewicka, M. (2010). What makes neighborhood different from home and city? Effects of place scale on place attachment. *Journal of Environmental Psychology, 30*(1), 35–51.
Lynnebakke, B., & Aasland, A. (2022). Striking roots: Place attachment of international migrants, internal migrants and local natives in three Norwegian rural municipalities. *Journal of Rural Studies, 94*, 488–498.
Maharaj, P. (2013). *Aging and health in Africa*. Springer.
Manzoni, C., & Rolfe, H. (2019). Older people in migration: The grey areas of the refugee crisis. *Journal of Ethnic and Migration Studies, 45*(4), 595–611.
Moyo, I. (2018). Migration, health, and integration: Exploring the experiences of older migrants in South Africa. *Journal of Ethnic and Migration Studies, 44*(8), 1295–1313.
Murray, S. (2019). From "state of emergency" to the ordinary: Lived citizenship in post-apartheid South Africa. *Journal of Southern African Studies, 45*(1), 3–21.
Nisa, C. F., B'elanger, J. J., & Schumpe, B. M. (2020). On solid ground: Secure attachment promotes place attachment. *Journal of Environmental Psychology, 70*, 101463.
Oyebamiji, I. S. (2021). *Life across borders: A case study of Nigerian immigrant women in Durban, South Africa*. Unpublished doctoral dissertation. University of KwaZulu-Natal.
Oyebamiji, S. I. (2023). Innovation and flexibility: Nigerian women in Durban's informal economy. In P. Maharaj (Ed.), *Migrant traders in South Africa*. Palgrave Macmillan.
Phillimore, J., & Goodson, L. (2017). Problem or opportunity? Asylum seekers, ageing and social policy in the UK. *Social Policy and Society, 16*(2), 213–228.
Scannell, L., & Gifford, R. (2014). The psychology of place attachment. In R. Gifford (Ed.), *Environmental psychology: Principles and practice* (5th ed.). Optimal Books.

Sieng, V., & Szabo, A. (2023). Exploring the place attachments of older migrants in Aotearoa: A life course history approach. *Advances in Life Course Research, 57*, 100560.

United Nations. (2019). *World population ageing 2019: Highlights*. Department of Economic and Social Affairs, Population Division, United Nations.

Warnes, A. M., Friedrich, K., Kellaher, L., Torres, S., & Walsh, K. (Eds.). (2016). *Environment and ageing: Environmental contexts and older people's well-being*. Routledge.

Williams, C. (2018). Economic hardships and resilience of older migrants: A qualitative study. *International Journal of Social Welfare, 27*(2), 131–140.

World Health Organization (WHO). (2002). *Active ageing: A policy framework*. WHO.

World Health Organization (WHO). (2015). *World report on ageing and health*. WHO.

World Health Organization (WHO). (2022). *Ageing and health*. WHO.

Zihindula, G., Maharaj, P., & Dunn, S. (2023). No protection, no support: Older migrants operating in South Africa's informal economy. In P. Maharaj (Ed.), *Migrant traders in South Africa*. Palgrave Macmillan.

11

Architectural Design as a Response to the Elderly

Viloshin Govender

Abstract As the population ages, architecture needs to respond to the needs of the elderly. The design of buildings, public spaces and homes can significantly impact the health, well-being and quality of life of the elderly. Universal design in architecture refers to a design approach that aims to create spaces, buildings and products that can be used by as many people as possible, regardless of age, size, ability or mobility. By responding to the needs of the elderly, architecture can help create a more supportive and inclusive environment for people of all ages. This chapter explores how architecture can create a more supportive environment for the elderly. It goes beyond pragmatic issues, showing that the design of buildings, public spaces and homes should prioritise accessibility, safety and mobility and incorporate features that promote social interaction, relaxation and overall health. The environment should be inclusive, accommodating and accessible for all, including the elderly.

V. Govender (✉)
School of Built Environment and Development Studies, University of KwaZulu-Natal, Durban, South Africa
e-mail: GovenderV3@ukzn.ac.za

P. Maharaj (ed.), *Navigating Ageing in South Africa*, Sustainable Development Goals Series, https://doi.org/10.1007/978-981-97-9088-3_11

Keywords Lost spaces • Built environment • Inclusive • Resilient • African cities

Introduction

In South Africa, the ever-growing elderly population is increasing the need for an appropriate design and alternate forms of retirement. According to the Global Retirement Index conducted in 2015, retirement security is assessed in terms of material well-being, health, finances in retirement and quality of life. South Africa is ranked amongst the worst countries in the world regarding retirement with very few options available to the elderly (Marx, 2016).

Public spaces, including parks, sidewalks and other outdoor spaces, should also be designed with the elderly in mind. Outdoor spaces should be designed with non-slip surfaces, benches for resting and plenty of shade. Sidewalks should be wide enough to accommodate wheelchairs and walkers, and crosswalks should be marked with visible signage. In addition to physical features, architecture can also respond to the psychological needs of the elderly. For example, creating social spaces that encourage interaction can help combat loneliness and social isolation. Public spaces can be designed with benches, picnic tables and other seating options that encourage people to gather and interact. In residential buildings, communal areas such as lounges and community kitchens can facilitate greater social interaction.

Architecture can also respond to the environmental needs of the elderly. For example, incorporating green spaces and natural elements into the design of buildings and public spaces can help promote relaxation and reduce stress. Access to green spaces can also encourage physical activity and improve overall health. Elderly empowerment spaces refer to environments specifically designed to empower and support older adults. These spaces are designed for older adult's unique needs and abilities, promoting independence, safety and social interaction. Retirement homes and elderly shelters found in Durban often ignore the concept of empowerment, and they are designed to isolate the elderly from society.

Current retirement facilities cater exclusively to the economically empowered in society. Although these facilities respond to some needs of the elderly through universal design principles that cater to their physical needs, vital social integration needs are ignored, leaving the elderly without a meaningful sense and purpose. Socialisation, sense of belonging, and life satisfaction of the elderly can help prevent cognitive decline in elderly individuals (Dinçer et al., 2023).

Institutions, old-age homes and retirement villages are support mechanisms and care facilities for elderly individuals and their families. However, it is often viewed as a gated community, with little or no interaction with the outside. The elderly's role in society is often negatively or positively perceived. Positively, as active members of society, based on culture as leaders, they are often held in high regard and seen as primary caregivers. Negatively, as those in poor health, diminishing mental ability, negative personality traits, lonely and unable to be financial contributors (Marx, 2016). Old-age homes, retirement and nursing homes are typically located in suburban areas, consisting of a single-room, dormitory-style designs, catering to basic needs. These environments often do not replicate the feeling of a home and are cold, sterile, and clinical spaces in which the elderly are forced to spend the remaining years of their life.

A new approach needs to be conceptualised, where the elderly can be integrated into society through shared spaces that can promote intergenerational sustainability. This approach can be a viable solution to promote social togetherness and allow the elderly to gain a sense of meaning and purpose. Theories and concepts such as Martin Heidegger's place-making, Kenneth Frampton's critical regionalism, Christian Norberg-Schulz's architecture and space, and Juhani Palasmaa's sensory perception go beyond the static homogenous designs in dealing with the elderly, allowing elderly care facilities to respond to more than just their physical needs, but also their mental well-being and self-esteem. Most centres for the elderly are inadequately equipped in fulfilling their needs. Although most do provide support in some ways, there is little consideration of psychological, physical and social needs. Homes for the aged are often associated with institutionalisation, creating a negative outlook amongst the elderly and isolating them from society. Therefore, a more meaningful architecture for the elderly is needed, one that addresses their social, psychological and physical needs that foster a more caring and inclusive environment.

Conceptualising Homes for the Elderly

In urban settings devoid of cultural richness and significance, inhabitants often experience a profound sense of detachment. As environments shape individuals, so too do individuals shape their environments, as noted by Lynch (1960), who observed that people develop personal connections with different aspects of their city based on accumulated memories and meanings over time. Two concepts are pivotal in understanding cultural memory: 'communicative' or 'everyday memory', which lacks distinct cultural attributes, and collective self-image, which is informed by individual recollections. This notion resonates strongly in places like elderly care facilities, where residents often lack a sense of belonging. Typically, introduced to these spaces during times of transition due to illness or an inability to live independently, the elderly often find themselves in environments devoid of personal significance or attachment.

To foster a sense of belonging, individuals, regardless of age, require a connection to their surroundings and society at large (Dovey, 1985). Human beings have perpetually moulded their environments to meet their needs, particularly those that underpin values, significance and a sense of engagement. Social scientist Robert Morey delineates these fundamental human needs, which include the requirement for external energy and stimuli, bodily conditions conducive to habitual responses, and predictable, favourable surroundings (Morey, 1940).

When these needs are unmet, individuals experience turmoil and unease, prompting them to exert control over their environment. Consequently, the built environment plays a crucial role in fulfilling human needs and enriching human life. Whether natural or constructed, an individual's immediate environment profoundly influences their psychology, with elements such as form, scale, proportion, colour and materials, impacting mood.

In the context of elderly care facilities, individual living spaces are designed to cater to basic needs, offering residents autonomy in maintaining personal hygiene and preparing meals. However, despite efforts to incorporate universal design principles, these spaces often lack a sense of belonging, as they tend to adhere to generic layouts that overlook contextual relevance.

Communal areas within these facilities serve as informal spaces for socialisation but face architectural challenges related to placement within urban environments, access to amenities, social interaction, accessibility, sensory experience, comfort, safety and security. Furthermore, many care facilities have been designed with an exclusive demographic in mind based on social, racial, economic and age-related criteria. As such, they often fail to address the diverse needs of society. Therefore, it is imperative that these facilities adapt to the local context and incorporate inclusive design principles to better serve their inhabitants and foster a sense of belonging within their communities.

Universal Design as a Response Towards the Elderly

Universal design aims to make life easier for all users, by creating friendlier and healthier spaces by placing the elderly and physically disabled on an equal playing field. Universal design draws on architectural and accessibility standards, coupled with design principles that integrate accessibility principles into design responses.

Problems experienced by disabled people in using the built environment have been recognised by the South African Human Rights Council (SAHRC) and go beyond physical disabilities to include visually impaired users and those with mental disabilities. It also includes ageing disability. In South Africa, the disability policy has been implemented in the form of the South African National Standards policy, particularly in Part T of the SANS 10400, focusing on facilities for persons with disabilities and Part T of the SANS 10400, focusing on fire protection in the built environment. This policy regulates all professionals in the built environment to take measures to create universally accessible and barrier-free environments to a diversity of users' needs.

The benefits of universal design for the elderly are immense. A universally designed environment can adapt to the changing needs of a user throughout their lifetime, allowing users to live in their homes and communities and to age in place. The negative outcomes of relocating due to the need for assisted living facilities for the elderly, results in social relationships being severed because of relocation and loss of independence (Campbell, 2016).

Universal design was first pioneered by Ron Mace, a wheelchair-using architect, who developed principles that advocated for accessible environments for all. The seven recognised principles of universal design are:

1. Equitable use, providing the same means of use for all users, avoiding stigmatising users.
2. Flexibility in use, a design that is accommodating to a wide range of abilities and disabilities.
3. Simple and intuitive, making sure the design is easy to understand, regardless of the user's knowledge and skill level.
4. Perceptible information, a design that communicates effortlessly to all users regardless of the ambient condition or sensory ability of the users.
5. Tolerance and error, designs that minimise hazards.
6. Low physical effort, the design can be used easily without creating fatigue in users.
7. Size and approach for users, appropriate size in relation to the user, using clear sight lines and appropriately placed seating elements.

These principles recognise that everyone will experience a period of reduced sensory, physical or intellectual disability in their lifetime (Jackson, 2013). In order to create active lifestyles for the elderly, the environment needs to be designed for universal access. Barriers such as level changes (stairs), long corridors, and poorly designed outdoor spaces inhibit the elderly from engaging in physical activities in their daily routines. This leads to sedentary behaviour, mental ill-health and cognitive decline (Ahrentzen & Tural, 2015).

For the elderly, universal design elements go beyond including ramps over the use of stairs and look at details that make their daily lives easier. Examples can be found in hallways designed with a minimum width of 1.8 m to allow users in wheelchairs to pass each other easily, designing cupboards to be lower to avoid strain when reaching for items or having parking widths that are wider so that the elderly can easily come in and out of cars.

These interventions are not costly and are seen as add-ons to a building. They are implemented at the design phase and allow the building to adapt to users' needs over time. This approach to design allows the built environment to respond to the specific needs of the elderly at the same time promoting active lifestyles and physical activities.

The Phenomenology of Space for the Elderly

Extensive literature and research underscore the significance of healing and restorative environments in shaping patients' experiences positively. Phenomenology theory emphasises the importance of sensory design in crafting architectural spaces that offer profound experiential impact. Psychologists have delved into the architectural realm, examining elements such as movement, shapes, music, colour contrast, geometric illusions, patterns and their correlation with human emotions and experiences. This exploration resonates with Gestalt theory, which elucidates individuals' interpretations of their surroundings, encompassing space, objects and other people (Mistrey, 2011). Phenomenological theorists like Alberto Perez-Gomaez, Peter Zumthor, and Steven Holl advocate for architectural designs that prioritise the human experience and its stimuli.

Crucially, life events, daily stressors, social support systems and coping mechanisms significantly influence depressive symptoms (Gory et al., 1990). Similarly, the elderly may have to contend with depressive symptoms stemming from traumatic life experiences and detachment from social structures and the built environment, as noted by Gory et al. (1990).

Architecture profoundly impacts individuals' senses and perceptions, serving as a conduit for understanding the surrounding environment.

Pallasmaa (2005) posits that the human body serves as the locus of perception, thought and consciousness, with the senses playing a pivotal role in articulating, storing and processing sensory responses and cognition. Pallasmaa (2005) emphasises the imperative of considering the interplay of senses in architectural design, critiquing contemporary societies for overemphasis on visual aesthetics at the expense of other sensory experiences, which fosters detachment.

The physical environment exerts a tangible influence on individual's physical and psychological well-being. Surfaces and textures allow individuals to tangibly connect with their environment, eliciting sensory responses. Auditory stimuli, such as the tranquillity of falling water or the cacophony of urban traffic, profoundly affect individual's emotional states. Architecture can manipulate auditory sensations to induce tranquillity, fostering calmness and meditation. Similarly, scents and tastes evoke memories, imbuing spaces with emotional resonance. The interplay of senses is pivotal in shaping individual's well-being, as the environment can modulate both psychological and physical states, influencing mood and mental health outcomes.

The sterile environments prevalent in many elderly care facilities engender a sense of alienation, severing ties to the familiar and comfort of home. The resultant lack of connection and orientation exacerbates psychological distress among the elderly. Architectural environments wield the power to heal, as they engage both the physical and psychological senses. To rehabilitate the psychological well-being of the elderly, spaces must foster a sense of connection and meaning, stimulating all senses. Pallasmaa (2005) advocates for environments where individuals feel integrated rather than isolated, underscoring the importance of sensory stimulation. Norberg-Schulz's concept of genius loci complements Pallasmaa's phenomenology, focusing on the micro-level to evoke a sense of place while also considering the broader environmental context.

Towards the Creation of Meaningful Spaces for the Elderly: Genius Loci

Genius loci, coined by Norberg-Schulz (1980), encapsulates a location's distinctive essence, often described as its 'spirit of place'. Introduced to architectural discourse by Norberg-Schulz and later embraced by post-modernists, this concept celebrates the inherent charm found in the harmony between human culture and nature within a space. Unlike planned environments, the spirit of place emerges organically, driven by the innate need for shelter, resulting in spaces imbued with unique character and identity.

Norberg-Schulz's (1980) exploration of genius loci aims to illuminate people's experiential engagement with their physical surroundings and society's cultural interpretation of space. He expands the concept beyond mere physical location, incorporating elements such as earth, sky and natural landscapes into the notion of place. In contrast, Trancik's space theory (1986) emphasises the cultural and human dimensions that imbue space with meaning, transforming it into a place within a specific cultural context (Tickley, 2011).

Kevin Lynch's concept of place further enriches our understanding by identifying elements such as paths, edges, landmarks, districts and nodes as key reference points within a space. These elements form the basis of cultural systems of orientation, shaping individuals' perceptions of their environment and fostering a sense of connection and familiarity. Architecture, as Lynch suggests, has the potential to heal, particularly in the context of the elderly, by addressing both physical and psychological needs. By incorporating design principles that prioritise context, local materials and socio-cultural factors, architects can create spaces that not only promote health and well-being but also celebrate the inherent genius loci of the site.

It is incumbent upon architects to adapt architectural styles to produce contextually responsive and responsible designs, ensuring the provision of comfortable and healthy environments for the elderly. By embracing sensory realism through architecture, the elderly can be afforded a unique and enriching experience, fostering a sense of empowerment and self-worth. In countering placeless and meaningless environments, care facilities must prioritise healing and rehabilitation, fostering connections, independence and transitions that empower the elderly within their built environment.

Methodological Approach—Describing Analysis Methods

This chapter is based on archival and empirical research. The archival research consisted of the literature review related to elderly housing and elderly care facilities as well as the architecture of elderly homes, places and universal design. The empirical research consisted of questionnaires, interviews and case studies conducted by postgraduate students on topics dealing with architecture and the elderly. The research was conducted in various facilities that cater for people aged 60 years and over within the Durban CBD, between 2015 and 2017.

Mapping Care Existing Care Facilities for the Elderly

One of the main elderly housing facilities located in Durban is The Association for the Aged (TAFTA). TAFTA was established in 1958 in Durban. Their mission statement promotes the well-being of the elderly in order to alleviate distress of the elderly and vulnerable groups. TAFTA is a registered NPO, which is dedicated to providing homes and support facilities for the elderly. Through a partnership with the Department of Social Development (DSD), services such as suitable accommodation and social support services are provided for the elderly. TAFTA currently owns 14 buildings in the Durban Metropolitan area and provides accommodation for 5500 people. TAFTA is available to the elderly over the age of 60 and provides accommodation for the frail elderly through frail care units and assisted living units. The following precedents were analysed for their architectural response towards the elderly (Fig. 11.1).

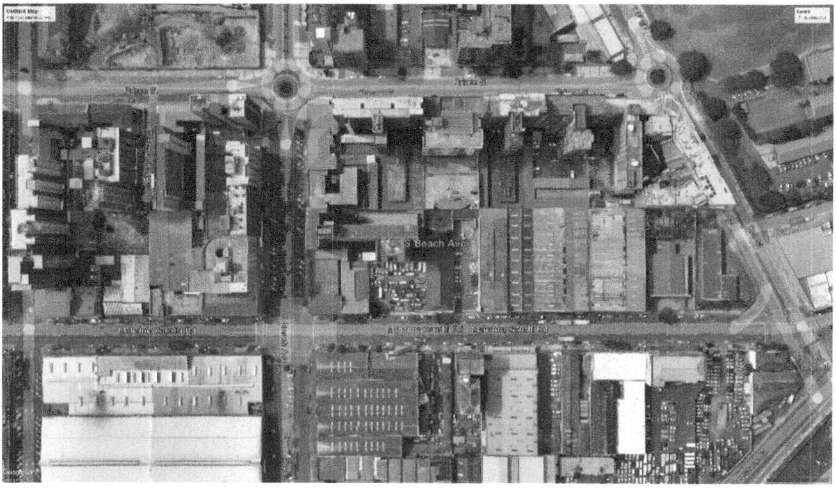

Fig. 11.1 TAFTA Lodge 42 South Beach Avenue, Durban. Source: www.earth.google.com

TAFTA Lodge is located at 42 South Beach Avenue, Durban, TAFTA on Ridge and TAFTA Cambridge Gardens. These precedents were analysed according to their services provided, functions and response to the elderly needs.

TAFTA Lodge is located at 42 South Beach Avenue, Durban, and is in a mixed-use residential area. The location is close to the South Beach Node and next to the Ushaka marine world. This is ideal as it is close to leisure activities for the elderly. The building typology is a block of flats with 203 units, 51 being dedicated to couple/co-sharing and 152 for single-unit typologies. Each living unit is self-contained with a small bedroom, lounge/dining area, small kitchen and bathroom. Rooms are decorated according to the user's preference, filling it with picture frames and furniture from their homes. This helps create a sense of belonging and familiarity for them (Fig. 11.2).

Communal features include a common lounge and dining area, with a kitchen servicing both. Amenities such as hair salons, tuck shops and laundry facilities are also found on site. One of the biggest drawbacks of the facility is the lack of green spaces with access to the outside. This has forced the walkways to become spaces for social interaction. Although

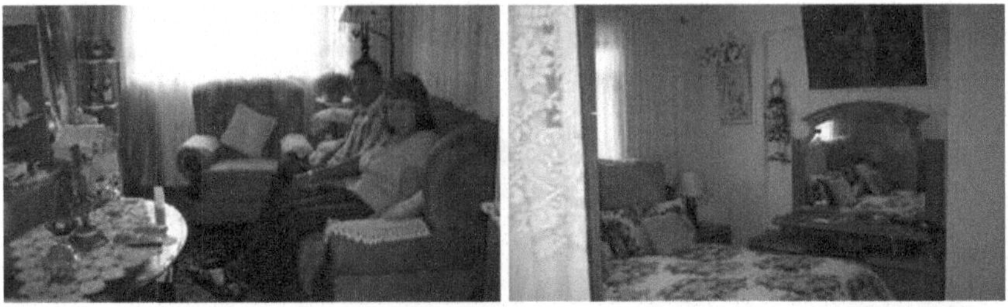

Fig. 11.2 Interior spaces and room decoration at TAFTA Lodge. Source: Marx (2016)

the spaces in the bedrooms are decorated to the user's preference, the overall feel of the building is institutionalised. Marx (2016) states that residences were warm and inviting, but it was clear that there was also a sense of loneliness and isolation experienced by the residents.

Long narrow hallways and no meeting spaces for family visits or reception areas create a sense of disorientation. Not having clear pathways or signage in a building adds to the sense of confusion, especially amongst the elderly. The lack of greenery in the building also adds to the creation of a cold and uninviting environment, with no sense of place. Some notable activities found at TAFTA South Beach are:

- Skills training,
- Self-defence training, fire training and financial planning,
- Meals on wheels,
- Social clubs, bingo, bridge and dancing,
- Assistance from social workers (Fig. 11.3).

TAFTA Cambridge Gardens is located at 130 North Ridge Road, Morningside. This facility accommodates 77 units with multiple living situations. This facility is within a residential neighbourhood, allowing for green spaces and gardens to occur within its linear block design. The outdoor spaces have ample seating and are well vegetated, aiding in a sense of place being created. Common facilities include a hair salon and tuck shop. The block sizes of the residential units do not respond to the human scale, creating a dominating effect for the user.

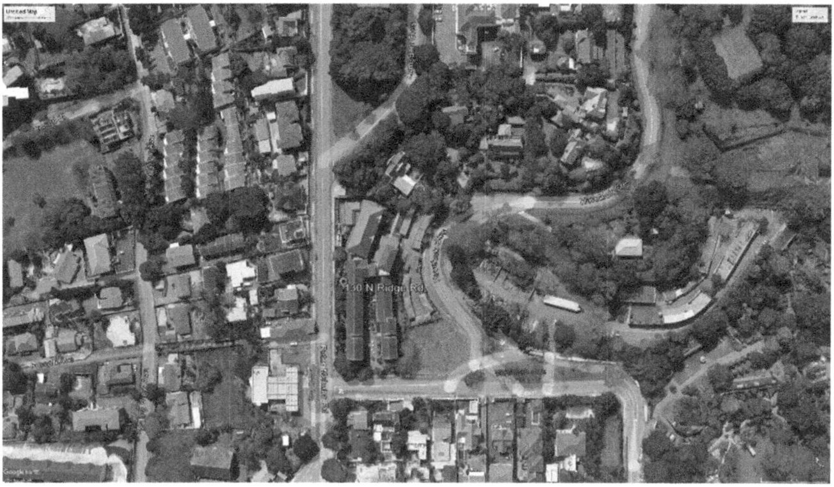

Fig. 11.3 TAFTA Cambridge Gardens: 130 North Ridge Road, Durban. Source: www.earth.google.com

TAFTA on Ridge is located at 51 East Street in Overport. This building is situated in a residential area, surrounded by mixed-use neighbourhoods. The facility has assisted living (48 units) and independent living units (110 units) and sits next to a public park. Internal corridors of the facility contrast starkly to the exterior spaces, with corridors being poorly lit. This is due to the corridors being double loaded, with units on both sides, blocking natural light from entering. Common spaces are located on the ground floor, with visual connections to the garden spaces (Fig. 11.4).

Common lounges serve as co-mingling spaces, residents use these spaces as an access to the garden as well. The building's exterior façade creates a sense of industrialisation; this is due to standard window sizes being used, red face bricks and concrete being used as façade elements that all create a harsh and cold experience of the building. This in turn creates a lack of identity for the users who cannot connect with the building as it lacks a sense of place.

Amenities found on site include:

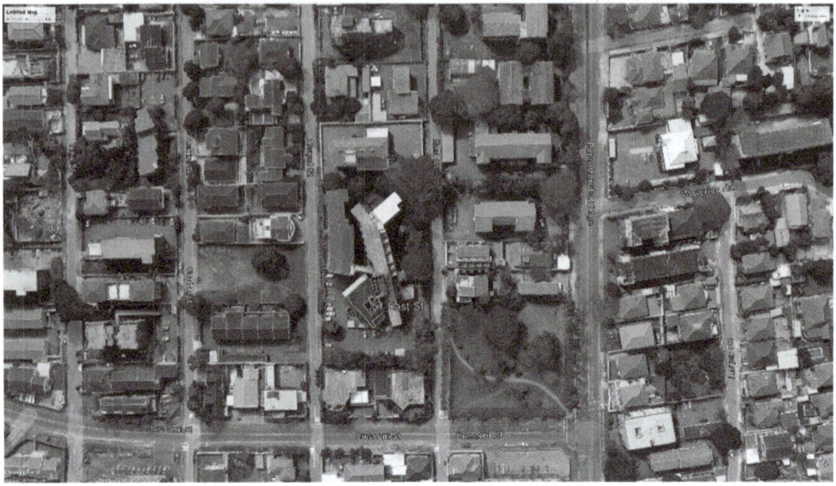

Fig. 11.4 TAFTA on Ridge: 51 East Street in Overport, Durban. Source: www.earth.google.com

- Weekly clinics,
- Home-based care services,
- Lounge with television,
- Library,
- Garden with aviary,
- Coin-operated washing machines.

The analysis of existing elderly care facilities revealed some positives and negatives of design considerations that affect the elderly. Some features found in the analysis are practicality (ease of access), comfort (creating a homely feel), use of natural light for healing, open plan space promoting views, use of greenery and flexible communal spaces. Openness can be translated to creating transparency and allowing the elderly to be seen, negating the effects of feeling isolated. Uncluttered, open spaces can also aid in creating a sense of calm amongst the elderly, as a space that promotes tranquillity.

Findings from questionnaires conducted by Omarjee (2013) and Marx (2016) reveal that bedroom sizes are not a problem for residents; rather, circulation is a concern, and wheelchair and stroller access becomes challenging when using passages. Greenery incorporated into the design is particularly important for the elderly as it can aid in the healing process as well as provide extracurricular activities for the elderly. The corridor is seen as the main design element that should be enhanced. This is a social space in the building and allows residents to meet their fellow residents. The corridors analysed in most TAFTA buildings have no natural light and sitting spaces within the corridors (Fig. 11.5).

Figure 11.6a shows a typical layout found in the case studies of TAFTA accommodations. This type of arrangement does not promote communal living or integrate vegetation and nature into the layout design; the walkway does not allow for natural lighting to create the feeling of home. Figure 11.6b on the other hand can be used as a design alternative, allowing for natural lighting and communal space, creating the feeling of a 'neighbourhood'.

The finding revolves around the analysis of three elderly housing facilities under TAFTA in Durban, South Africa: TAFTA Lodge, TAFTA Cambridge Gardens and TAFTA on Ridge. These facilities provide accommodation and support services for the elderly, catering to their needs through various amenities and living arrangements.

TAFTA Lodge, situated near leisure activities in a mixed-use residential area, offers self-contained units decorated according to residents' preferences. However, drawbacks include a lack of green spaces, leading to social spaces being confined to narrow hallways. Loneliness and isolation are reported among residents, highlighting the importance of communal areas and outdoor access.

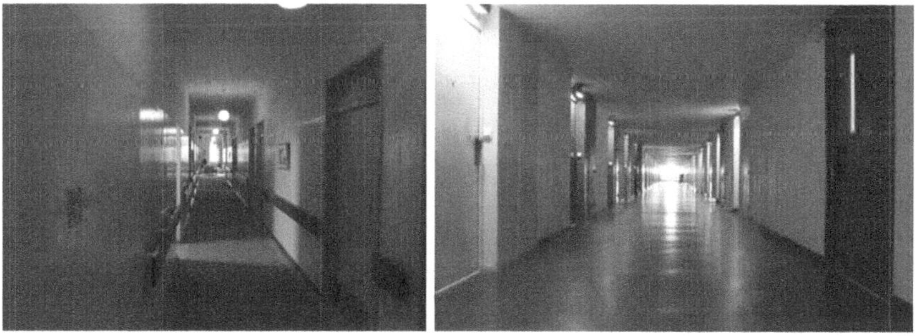

Fig. 11.5 Interior corridor views at TAFTA on Ridge. Source: Omarjee (2013)

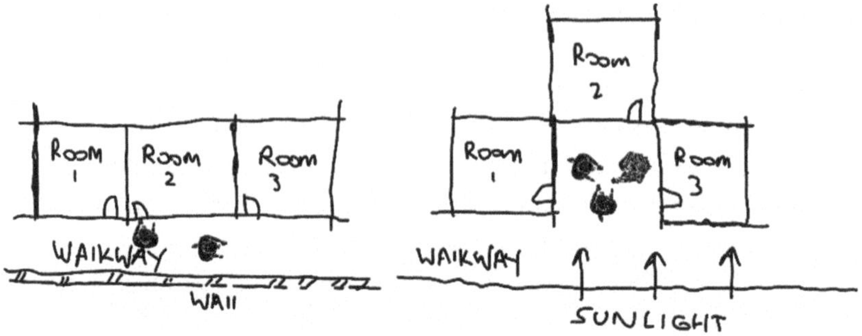

Fig. 11.6 (**a**) and (**b**): Room layout sketches

TAFTA Cambridge Gardens, located within a residential neighbourhood, provides ample green spaces and gardens, contributing to a sense of place. However, the block sizes of residential units may overshadow the human scale, potentially affecting resident's comfort.

TAFTA on Ridge, situated in a mixed-use neighbourhood next to a public park, offers both assisted and independent living units. While common spaces connect visually to garden areas, the building's industrialised facade and lack of natural light in corridors create a cold atmosphere, impacting resident's sense of identity and place.

Overall, the analysis emphasises the importance of practicality, comfort and access to natural light and greenery in designing elderly care facilities. Open, uncluttered spaces can promote tranquillity and reduce feelings of isolation, while corridors should be enhanced to serve as social hubs with natural light and seating areas. Additionally, incorporating greenery into design not only aids in healing but also provides recreational opportunities for residents. Addressing circulation concerns, such as wheelchair access, is essential for ensuring resident's comfort and mobility within the facilities.

Exploring Proposed Elderly Care Facility Designs

The following architectural proposals were analysed as an architectural response to the elderly. Design proposals involved investigating existing elderly facilities and creating an appropriate architectural response based on case studies, interviews and questionnaires. The following criteria were highlighted as issues from the case study analysis: room design, common spaces, social interaction spaces, wayfinding, accessibility and facilities. When analysing the student responses, it is noted that the need for socialisation formed the focus of spatial design responses, with some allowing for intergenerational approaches to the architecture (Fig. 11.7).

The first proposal analysed unit typology designs. This deviated significantly from the TAFTA examples as it created an adaptive approach to the design. This allows users to accommodate family members, share spaces, and co-living units. This approach allows for multi-generational living, enabling the elderly to live with their families or have the option to adapt the space to their needs. Universal design has also been approached through the design of a wheelchair-friendly unit, which could be placed on the ground floor for ease of access. Important elements of the room design are to also include a balcony to serve as a connection to the outside. One key attribute to be considered is the design of the shower, not to include a step; this would be an easy way for the elderly to trip and fall, so walk-in showers are preferred.

Figure 11.8 highlights the connection to nature in the room layout design. This promotes an active lifestyle for the elderly with access to

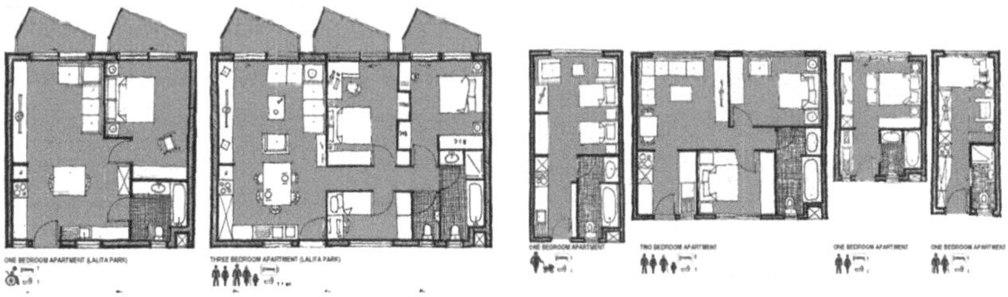

Fig. 11.7 Room layout typologies. Source: Mahadew (2018)

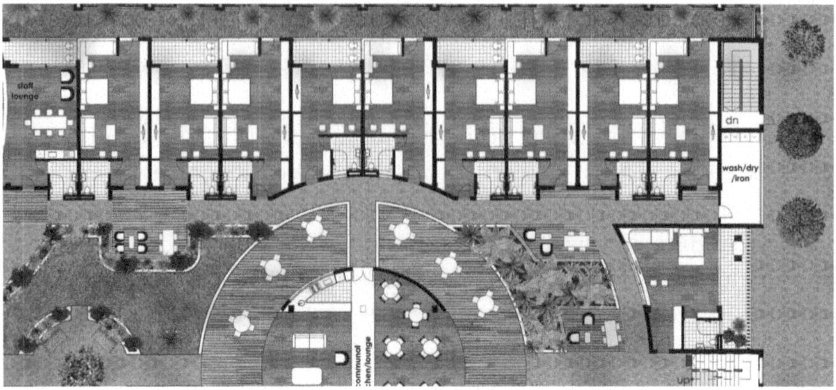

Fig. 11.8 Room layout typologies. Source: Omarjee (2013)

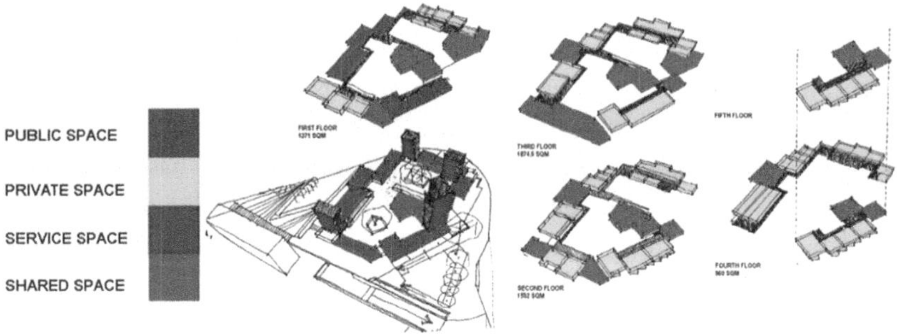

Fig. 11.9 Room layout typologies. Source: Mahadew (2018)

green and social spaces. The positive effects of outdoor spaces on the health of the elderly are emphasised by the open and semi-open spaces that directly interact with nature. Nature can be seen as a healing element, and incorporating this in the design through windows that open to garden views, porches, walkways with greenery and social spaces in gardens will help create a sense of place for the elderly. Figure 11.8 above also highlights degrees of privacy in the design; the elderly have private spaces in their rooms and social spaces as soon as they step out; this helps combat feelings of isolation, which the elderly in TAFTA lodges experience.

Figure 11.9 shows the distribution of spaces along movement paths. Creating public and private spaces on each floor can develop a sense of community instead of a dormitory feel. As highlighted in the example of the TAFTA lodges, the corridors are used as meeting spaces and pause spaces, as in some cases, there are no external relaxation spaces. Creating shared spaces allows the elderly to form bonds with each other, creating a neighbourhood feel. Service spaces such as lifts and stairs should be placed at central locations so that private rooms are easily accessible and identifiable by them.

Figure 11.10 highlights the concepts of Fig. 11.6b, using social space integrated into the corridor design layouts. By alternating the room layout, space is able to be created on the walkway. This form of shared space promotes bonds to be created as well as a sense of community. In high-density developments, where residents have no access to the ground floor spaces, recreation spaces can be achieved on the walkway spaces. The walkway space is also a type of space, forming part of the social sphere and has positive impacts on the elderly.

The inclusion of multi-generational spaces and co-mingling spaces as shown in Fig. 11.11 allows for intergenerational interaction to occur, including formal and informal interaction. These activities allow interaction from the broader community to strengthen ties and promote active participation. Strong visual links to these spaces would allow for constant activity and energy to be shared with the elderly, combating the sense of isolation (Fig. 11.12).

Elevations show an interaction between the exterior and interior spaces. The windows used in the building are not only for natural ventilation and lighting but also allow for a transition between natural elements

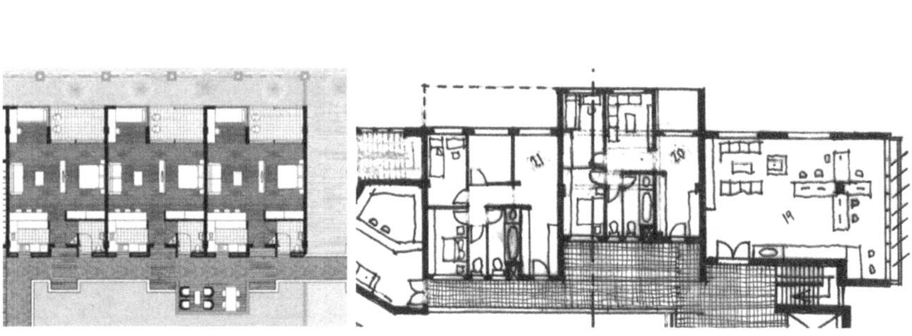

Fig. 11.10 Room layout typologies. Source: Omarjee (2013); Mahadew (2018)

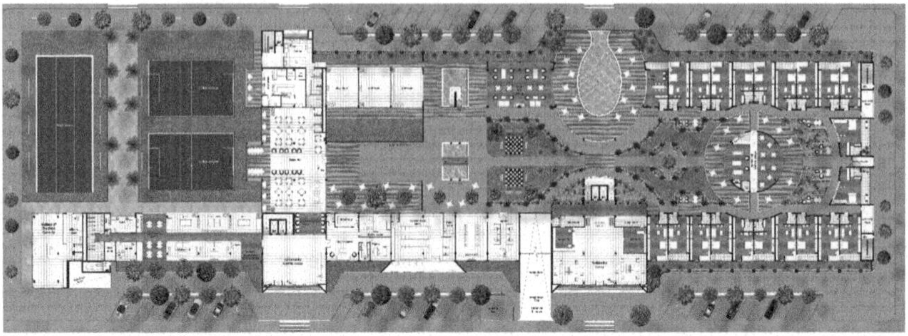

Fig. 11.11 Intergenerational facilities. Source: Omarjee (2013)

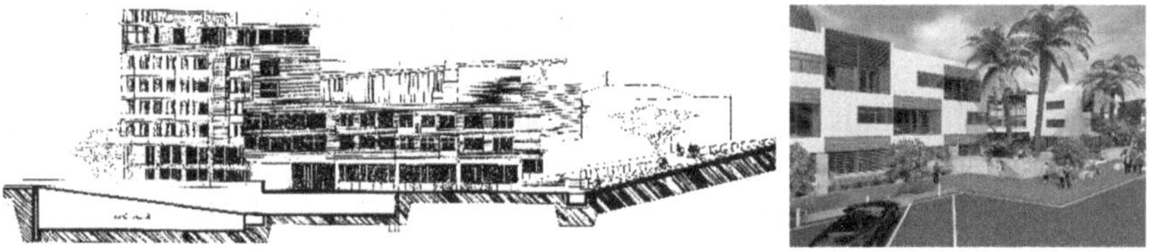

Fig. 11.12 Elevation analysis. Source: Omarjee (2013); Mahadew (2018)

and built form. Some spaces open to lush private courtyards, allowing for meditation, reflection and relaxation. The openness of fenestration on the façade also promotes active surveillance, which is important to the safety of the residents.

The analysis drawing on research on architectural responses to the needs of the elderly unveils several key insights. Through investigation and case study analysis of existing facilities for the elderly, this chapter underscores critical criteria including room design, common spaces, social interaction areas, wayfinding, accessibility and facilities.

The design responses showcased a departure from traditional approaches, with a notable emphasis on fostering socialisation and multigenerational living. By incorporating adaptable unit typologies and universal design principles, the architecture not only accommodates the needs of the elderly but also facilitates intergenerational cohabitation. This innovative approach not only promotes familial bonds but also empowers the elderly to tailor their living spaces to their preferences, enhancing their sense of agency and well-being.

Moreover, the integration of nature within the architectural design emerges as a central theme, with outdoor spaces serving as vital components for promoting an active and healthy lifestyle among the elderly. By incorporating elements such as garden views, porches and walkways with greenery, the architecture creates a therapeutic environment that nurtures both physical and mental well-being. Furthermore, the research emphasises the importance of communal spaces in fostering a sense of community and combating feelings of isolation. Through strategic placement and design of shared spaces along movement paths, the architecture encourages social interaction and neighbourhood bonding, enriching the lives of the elderly residents.

In addition, the incorporation of multi-generational and co-mingling spaces underscores the commitment to promoting inclusivity and active participation within the broader community. By facilitating formal and informal interactions between different age groups, the architecture fosters connections and strengthens social ties, creating a vibrant and supportive living environment.

Overall, the design responses present a holistic architectural response that not only addresses the specific needs of the elderly but also celebrates their contributions to the community. Through innovative design strategies and a human-centred approach, the research sets a precedent for creating inclusive and age-friendly built environments that enhance the quality of life for all.

Conclusion

The increasing elderly population in South Africa necessitates a re-evaluation of existing retirement and care facilities to better cater to the diverse needs of this demographic group. Traditional retirement facilities often fail to address the holistic well-being of the elderly, focusing primarily on physical needs while neglecting vital aspects such as social integration and psychological fulfilment. As a result, many elderly individuals experience feelings of loneliness, isolation and a lack of purpose in these environments.

To address these shortcomings, a new approach to designing homes for the elderly is proposed, one that emphasises meaningful integration into society through shared spaces promoting intergenerational sustainability. Drawing on concepts such as place-making, critical regionalism, architecture and space, and sensory perception, architects can create environments that go beyond mere functionality to nurture the mental, emotional and social well-being of the elderly.

By incorporating elements such as adaptable unit typologies, universal design principles and ample access to nature, architects can create spaces that empower the elderly to maintain a sense of agency and independence while fostering connections with their families and communities. Communal spaces play a crucial role in combating feelings of isolation and promoting social interaction, while multi-generational spaces facilitate active participation and inclusivity within the broader community.

It is recommended that stakeholders involved in the design and development of elderly care facilities in South Africa adopt a more holistic approach that prioritises the well-being and dignity of the elderly. This involves:

- Embracing innovative design strategies that go beyond conventional models to create environments that are conducive to the physical, mental and social health of the elderly.
- Prioritising the incorporation of communal spaces and amenities that promote social interaction, engagement and a sense of belonging.
- Integrating nature into architectural design to provide therapeutic environments that support the overall well-being of the elderly.
- Emphasising the importance of multi-generational living and fostering connections between different age groups to create vibrant and inclusive communities.
- Conducting further research and collaboration with experts in fields such as gerontology, psychology, and architecture to continually improve and refine the design of elderly care facilities.

By implementing these recommendations, stakeholders can contribute to the creation of age-friendly environments that enhance the quality of life for the elderly in South Africa, ensuring that they can age with dignity, purpose and fulfilment.

References

Ahrentzen, S., & Tural, E. (2015). The role of building design and interiors in ageing actively at home. *Building Research & Information, 43*(5), 582–601.
Campbell, N. (2016). The why and how of redesigning retirement communities for aging in place. *Housing and Society, 43*(1), 34–49.
Dinçer, A., Temel, S., & Merve, S. (2023). *Elderly care Centres and architectural studio experience.* Paper presented at international conference on new horizons in education. Rome.
Dovey, K. (1985). Home and homelessness. In I. Altman & C. M. Werner (Eds.), *Home environments. Human behaviour and environment.* Springer.
Gory, M., Ritchey, F., & Mullis, J. (1990). Depression among the homeless. *Journal of Health and Social Behaviour, 31*(1), 87–102.
Jackson, M. (2013). Universal design- assisting accessibility. *Sanctuary: Modern Green Homes, 25*, 85–87.
Lynch, K. (1960). *The image of the city*. MIT Press.
Lynch, K. (1992). *Good city form*. MIT Press.
Mahadew, R. (2018) *A sustainable community within a sustainable district: A multigenerational development in Overport, Durban.* Unpublished Master's dissertation. University of KwaZulu-Natal.
Marx, F. (2016) *Exploring alternative residential care facilities for the intermediate elder: Towards a retirement facility in Warwick junction, Durban.* Unpublished Master's dissertation. University of KwaZulu-Natal.
McTavish, G. (2010). *An architectural interventionist approach to urban revitalisation: A proposed hotel for Durban waterfront.* Unpublished Master's dissertation. University of KwaZulu-Natal.
Mistrey, M. (2011). *Architectural psychology and its impact on child development: A proposed educational Facility for Physically Disabled Children, Durban.* Unpublished Master's dissertation. University of KwaZulu-Natal.
Morey, R. (1940). Basic needs of man in society. *The Journal of Educational Research, 34*(1), 1–14.

Norberg-Schulz, C. (1980). *Genius loci—Towards a phenomenology of architecture*. Academy Editions.

Omarjee, J. (2013). *Care for the elderly through meaningful architecture: A proposed intergenerational mixed-use development, Durban*. Unpublished Master's dissertation. University of KwaZulu-Natal.

Pallasmaa, J. (2005). *Eyes of the skin: Architecture and the senses*. Wiley-Academy.

Tickley, L. (2011). *Context as an architectural design generator: A proposed arts Centre in Durban, South Africa*. Unpublished Master's dissertation. University of KwaZulu-Natal.

Trancik, R. (1986). *Finding lost space: Theories of urban design*. Van Nostrand Reinhold.

Index

P. Maharaj (ed.), *Navigating Ageing in South Africa*, Sustainable Development Goals Series, https://doi.org/10.1007/978-981-97-9088-3_11

The manufacturer's authorised representative in the EU is Springer Nature Customer Service Centre GmbH, Europaplatz 3, 69115 Heidelberg, Germany. If you have any concerns regarding our products, please contact ProductSafety@springernature.com

Printed and bound by CPI Group (UK) Ltd, Croydon, CR0 4YY
01/10/2026
02225925-0001